Dear Terri,

I am blessed
to have met you!

Ivette Smith Jr

Kiss
Your
Fat
Good-bye

Kiss Your Fat Good-bye

Written Especially for Women

Lorette Simonet-Jones

Aroha Press

AROHA PRESS
1293 NW Wall St. Suite 57
Bend OR 97701

Library of Congress Catalogue Number: 97-95375
ISBN: 0-9658948-3-5

This book has been printed on recycled paper.

Printed in the U. S. A.

To my husband
and two children,
who have honored my dreams.

Contents

Introduction   ix

1. Diets Are Fairy Tales   1

2. Which Numbers Count   11

3. Exercise: What, When, Why and
         How Much   19

4. Nutrition: A Piece of Cake   33

5. Food Calories: The Good, Bad,
         & The Ugly   49

6. Master Your Environment   69

7. Telling the Truth   81

8. Twenty E-Z Lowfat Recipes   99

   Endnotes   111

Introduction

Welcome to *Kiss Your Fat Good-bye.* Whether this is the first health and fitness book you have read, which I doubt, or the one hundredth, I hope that it will further you along your path toward vitality and well-being.

At any given moment there are approximately 50 million Americans on a diet. Americans spend over 30 BILLION dollars annually on diet programs, diet foods, and diet gimmicks. Yet, countless studies indicate that 98% of those who do lose weight, regain all of it within two years. I used to ask clients how many times they'd been on a diet. These are a few of answers I heard -

"Dozens."

"I've lost track."

"You name the diet, I've been on it."

Many of these people lost 30, 50, even 100 pounds, by eating as little as 500 calories a day, receiving daily injections of herbal concoctions or ingesting high priced, prepackaged meals. Others had gone to further extremes by getting their jaws wired, stomachs stapled, or submitting to intestinal bypasses. What may be astonishing to you is that even *these* measures did not work.

Kiss Your Fat Good-bye, liberates you from the dieting myths and manipulations. It presents the aspects of health and fitness that you *want* to know, that you *need* to know in order to be healthy and fit. In Chapter One you meet Jane who embarks on the quintessential diet. You go through all her trials and tribulations and you witness and understand the reasons she fails. Chapter Two introduces you to the *numbers that count,* the first of a series of essential steps to successful health and fitness management.

These physiological numbers are those from which you build the foundation for a winning plan. Chapter Three not only convinces you that exercise is imperative to health and fitness, but it also helps you design your own personalized program. You find out how much you need to do to stay fit and exactly how to achieve that goal. A book on fitness and health would not be complete without a chapter on nutrition. This book makes nutrition as easy as pie. And, don't let *anyone* tell you that calories *don't count*. Chapter Five acquaints you with a unique and logical system for applying calories to your lifestyle. Without them, you lack critical information about how your food choices impact your weight. Chapter Six teaches you how to master your environment. Sorry, willpower went out with "chewing 20 times before each bite and eating on miniature plates." The seventh chapter is about discovering and reclaiming your truth. Haven't you lived long enough with the lies? In this chapter you learn to confront the belief systems that keep you from succeeding. You are guided along several exercises that help you get in touch with your ability to speak out and let go of destructive eating patterns. The final chapter brings you a collection of twenty quick and simple lowfat recipes.

My own journey began long before my first class in nutrition. When I was eight years old my father became terminally ill with cancer. I watched as this robust 6'2" 49-year old man wasted away to 90 pounds. His death catalyzed my determination to find out what caused this disease. It wasn't long afterward that I spotted an article in Reader's Digest about the relationship between cancer and diet. The article stated that Americans had a high incidence of colon cancer, whereas the Japanese had a high incidence of stomach and esophageal cancer. Japanese people eat lots of vegetables, which was thought to reduce their risk of colon cancer. But their high intake of smoked and pickled foods was thought to be the culprit in the esophageal and stomach cancer. Americans, on the other hand, eat plenty of red meats and little vegetables. Could this attribute to their high incidence of colon cancer? Years later this has been proven to be true. What the study failed to mention was that drinking alcohol and smoking cigarettes directly contribute to stomach and esophageal cancer. My father drank and smoked heavily and he died of stomach and esophageal cancer. What I secretly believed, yet found no documentation to support, was that my father's death was caused by a profound sense of despair, one which he anesthetized with alcohol.

I vowed, at an early age, to never become an alcoholic as my father had been, and to this promise I stayed true. Unfortunately, my addiction took on a different form. It began at the age of fourteen when I started my first diet. I thought that if only I was thinner, everything in my life would magically be "perfect." What I didn't realize then was that this aspiration to become "model" thin had more to do with my lack of self worth than it did with the size of my dress. What I truly craved was acknowledgement and love. But of this fact I was not consciously aware. I had no idea that engaging in a string of diets was my way of avoiding years of emotional pain. And this avoidance lead me down the deadly and painful road of an eating disorder.

It took many years of hard work to restore myself to physical health and mental well-being. Ironically, it was through this work that I triumphed and learned to love and accept myself. My goal in writing this book is to share with anyone else struggling with weight, health and body image issues, the wisdom, experience and hope I have been privileged to receive along the way of my journey.

1   Diets Are Fairy Tales

Once upon a diet, there was a woman named Jane, who lost over 50 pounds. She didn't lose the weight **once**, but many times over. The problem is that she also regained those 50 pounds again and again. Jane has been conditioned, over the years, to focus on, or rather, obsess about her weight. Currently 200, her weight has contributed to her high blood pressure, skyrocketing cholesterol, and increased fatigue. Jane feels hopeless and helpless over her problem. Even her physician doesn't know what to do. Yet, she continues to *act* cheerfully, avoiding her *real* feelings about her weight.

Although body weight is one indicator for health and fitness, some of the real indicators are blood cholesterol, blood pressure, muscle strength and flexibility, cardiovascular and pulmonary health, lean body tissue and even one's mental outlook. In this book you will learn how to get fit and healthy. And, losing weight will simply be a by-product of the skills, behaviors and procedures you will practice.

Unfortunately, Jane is more concerned about losing weight than she is about getting fit and healthy, and so, she is about to embark on yet *another* diet. She will begin on Monday. (Doesn't everyone start their diets on Monday?) This particular one she has found in her favorite women's magazine.

DAY 1

Breakfast: 1/2 grapefruit
1 piece dry toast
1 poached egg
coffee or tea

Lunch: Chef's salad with
diet dressing
1 slice French bread
1 medium apple

Dinner: 4 oz. baked chicken
1/2 cup broccoli
One small baked potato
with 1/2 T sour cream
1/2 cup nonfat frozen
yogurt

At first glance, it appears there is nothing wrong with this menu. It includes protein, starch and an assortment of fruits and vegetables. It contains approximately 1000 calories and 27 grams of fat. So, what is the problem?

For starters, this menu borders on starvation and would be nearly impossible to maintain on a long term basis. And, since Jane did not create the menu herself, she lacks knowledge of successful food planning. As a result, she remains dependent.

The Definition of Dieting

For the past fifty-some years, millions of Americans have engaged in a popular, yet unhealthy, method of losing weight known as dieting. Dieting, in the traditional sense of the word, means practicing two polarized behaviors: starving and overeating. And this pattern leads to one result - failure. Of those who **do** manage to lose weight, ninety-eight percent regain it all within a frustratingly short period of time.

Many diets recommend eating between 800 and 1000 calories a day. This is not only extremely difficult to accomplish, but nearly impossible to supply the body with all the vitamins, minerals and energy it needs to perform its functions. What most frequently happens when you eat such a restricted diet is that you feel fatigued and irritable.

By starving ourselves we activate a counter-productive response that causes our metabolism to slow down and use less energy. This built-in survival process prevented our more primitive ancestors from dying during naturally occurring famines. Most of us don't need to worry about famine in this country. Instead many of us simply starve ourselves voluntarily. In response to severe caloric reduction, our bodies actually *hold on* to fat and metabolize lean body tissue (organs like the heart and kidneys). When the ratio of muscle-to-fat declines, metabolic rate falls. This is one reason why women, who have suffered the effects of an onslaught of restrictive diets, gain weight more readily.

Posing against all this, Jane is very "successful" on her first day. She usually is, because to Jane, "success" means that she has followed her diet perfectly and has maintained a feeling of *control*. She proceeds with Day Two.

DAY 2

Breakfast:	1/2 banana 1 cup cold cereal 1/2 cup nonfat milk Coffee or tea, black
Lunch:	Open-faced tuna sandwich 1/2 cup Cole slaw 1/2 melon
Dinner:	3 oz. grilled pork chop 1/2 cup carrots 1/2 cup rice with 1 tsp. margarine
Snack:	4 cups popcorn

3

As Day Two draws to an end, Jane feels lightheaded, but this doesn't alarm her. She believes her lightheadedness indicates that she is doing something "right."

On the morning of Day Three, Jane decides to weigh herself. She steps on the scale cautiously, trying not to move the numbers too fast. To Jane's delight the scale shows a three-pound loss. She shakes her fists triumphantly and declares, "This diet is working!"

But, wait! Has Jane really lost three pounds?

"Of course," you reply, "the scale says so, and who argues with the scale?"

Ah! But the fact is, Jane has **not** lost three pounds of fat. At her present weight, Jane burns approximately 2200 calories per day. (You will learn more about this in Chapter Two.) For the past two days she has eaten roughly 1000 calories. If we subtract 1000 from 2200, we see she has burned 1200 calories per day, totaling 2400. It takes 3500 calories to burn <u>one</u> pound of fat. If we divide 2400 by 3500, the result is 2/3 of a pound of fat. The remaining two and one third pounds that shows up on the scale is water.

During the course of a day, the body either retains or releases water depending on such conditions as:

* The salt content of the foods eaten.
* The hormonal cycles of the body.
* A change in the amount of exercise one does.
* Dieting

When you diet, you restrict the intake of calories, which causes the body to release a considerable amount of water. This process, known as "diuresis," shows up on the scale as a loss - *water* loss, not fat loss. Unfortunately, Jane doesn't know this, and if anyone told her at this point, she probably wouldn't believe them. To Jane, the scale is the "diet god."

DAY 3

Breakfast:	1 orange 1/2 bagel w/ 1 T. jelly coffee
Lunch:	4 oz. burger 1/2 c. cottage cheese Lettuce & tomato 4 melba toast
Dinner:	6 oz. white fish (baked) 1/2 cup noodles with 1/2 T low-cal margarine and 2 T. Parmesan cheese 1/2 cup green beans 1 small dinner roll
Snack:	1 cup fresh strawberries 6 oz. lowfat milk

It is 8 o'clock at night on Day Three and Jane has succeeded in staying on her diet another day. But the day is not over yet. Her husband comes home with a pizza. Pepperoni with extra cheese - Jane's favorite. When he remembers that she is on a diet, he apologizes. He brings the pizza into the family room where she won't see him eating it. But the rich aroma permeates the house, and Jane envisions the melted cheese, the spicy pepperoni, and the crisply baked crust. Her mouth waters, and then like magic, the rationalizations begin:

"Just <u>one</u> slice can't hurt."
"I've <u>been</u> <u>so</u> good. I deserve it."
"I can't deprive myself <u>forever</u>."

Just as she is about to surrender, her daughter walks in, "So Mom, how's your diet going?" This jolts Jane back into reality. She remembers the three-pound loss (on the scale) and her willpower returns. Instead of eating pizza she decides to take a long relaxing bubble bath. Before she turns out the light to go to sleep, she congratulates herself for making it through another day.

The Facts:

Jane has eaten approximately 1100 calories on Day Three. This means she has deficited an additional 1100 calories which brings her deficit total to 3500 - exactly one pound of fat.

DAY 4

The sun is up and so is Jane. She hops on the scale, still exhilarated by her willpower from the day before. She estimates that, since she was "so good," she should have lost a few more pounds. But when the scale registers the same weight as the previous day, her enthusiasm plummets. "This can't be!" she shrieks. Frustrated, she skips breakfast and heads to work.

When she arrives at her office she sees a memo on her desk. It is a reminder about the business luncheon she is expected to attend. She wonders how she'll manage to stay on her diet at the luncheon.

Around ten o'clock she heads into the breakroom for a cup of coffee and notices that some generous soul (she would like to kill whoever it was) has brought in doughnuts. Jane grits her teeth, pours her coffee, and marches back to her office. At her desk, she can't keep her mind on work. A voice from the breakroom keeps calling her. It's the voice of the doughnuts. "You didn't eat any breakfast," the voice reminds her. "Just *one* can't hurt." She checks to see if anyone notices as she sneaks back into the breakroom.

She is relieved to find herself alone with three remaining doughnuts. There is an ancient myth known amongst dieters: "If no one sees you eating, it doesn't count." Within seconds one chocolate-glazed has passed through her lips. She finishes the last two before anyone comes in and licks the chocolate from her fingers.

As she heads back to her desk, she hears another voice. This time it is not as kind as the first. This time it is her own voice. "You've blown it. You are a failure." Her anger at and disappointment in herself are overwhelming. Instead of forgiving herself, (who ever does that?) she decides that today is a "failure" and she will start over *tomorrow*. This decision leaves the rest of the day wide open. During the business luncheon, she gobbles up the chicken, potatoes, peas, buttered roll and dessert.

After work she meets her husband at the movie theater. The smell of fresh popcorn fills her nostrils and she decides a medium bucket with a diet coke can't do any more damage than she has already done.

She goes to bed feeling defeated. She scolds herself, "How could I do that, especially after being so perfect for three days?" Before going on with the story, let's check in with the facts. Do Jane's feelings of "failure" match reality?

DAY 4	FOOD	CALORIES
	Three 2 oz. doughnuts	750
	Roasted chicken	350
	1/2 c potatoes w/ gravy	250
	Veggies with butter	150
	One dinner roll	150
	w/ butter	
	Apple cobbler	550
	w/ ice cream	
	Medium popcorn	300
	Total	2500

Remember, at her present weight, Jane burns 2200 calories. Therefore, on Day Four she has eaten 300 over her maintenance calories. But to Jane, it *feels* like she has eaten thousands more.

DAY 5

The next morning, after a rotten night's sleep, Jane drags herself from bed with a faint conviction that she will start her diet over. The bathroom scale, like a magnet, lures her. The last time she stood on her scale, it had registered a three-pound *loss*. Today, after falling from her diet, and eating popcorn loaded with salt, the scale shows a four-pound weight gain. She weighs one pound more than when she started!

A glance at the facts, in terms of "fat-versus-the-scale:"

Date	Scale	Cal. Deficited	Total Deficited
DAY 1	200 lb.	-1200	
DAY 2	197	-1200	-2400
DAY 3	197	-1100	-3500
DAY 4	197	+300	-3200
DAY 5	201		

Notice that Jane has deficited a total of 3200 calories. The four-pound gain on the scale is **water**, not fat.

The best way to rid the body of excess water is by drinking *more* water. Two quarts a day is recommended. This flushes out the areas between cells. Bloating dissipates naturally and healthy hydration is maintained. Unfortunately, most people would rather take a diuretic pill, which actually creates <u>more</u> bloating. Diuretics squeeze water from between the cells, temporarily relieving bloatedness, yet leaving cells dehydrated. As soon as the next drop of water comes their way, the cells soak up and retain it, causing more swelling.

Again, Jane does not know this. All she knows is that she feels depressed and defeated. Her feelings, though valid, are not based on facts. This is when the old tapes begin to play, "You will never be thin." "You are a failure." And it is these feelings that cause her to *act* as if she really <u>is</u> a failure.

On Day Five, Jane abandons the idea of losing weight - that is, at least until the next diet comes along. Once again, she becomes a victim of the dieting dilemma.

What <u>Does</u> Work?

Jane's method of depriving herself, using the number on the scale as the only barometer for success, and emotionally reacting to that number, is a surefire formula for failure. To achieve long-term fitness and health success, Jane needs to understand the facts about how metabolism, calories, nutrition and physical activity all work together. She must learn to incorporate specific skills and behaviors to generate positive results. She must also discover the underlying social and emotional issues that keep her trapped in destructive eating patterns. If your story is at all similar to Jane's, or if you simply want to become fit and healthy, continue reading.

2 Which Numbers Count?

There was a time, before I understood health and fitness, that I was perpetually strategizing to lose those notorious last ten pounds. I had become an expert at devising "thirty-day" menus. My master plan, usually a neatly drawn graph, projected the exact date I would achieve physical nirvana. Despite all my starving, sweat, and tears, I always fell short of my goal. Part of this was because, if I *had* succeeded, I would no longer have had something to obsess about. But the main reason was that, I, like Jane, was measuring my success on one number - the number on the scale.

Is "Ideal" Weight Really Ideal?

Although you may have worshipped it nearly every morning of your adult life, the scale is **not** the sole indicator of health and fitness success. Nor is it a symbol of one's physical value, or lack of it. Yet, tossing it is not necessarily the answer either. The scale converts your bones, fluids, muscles, organs and fat into a gross measurement of pounds we have come to know as our "weight."

One of the first things the doctor did the moment after you were born was to put you on a scale and record your weight. That weight was then compared to the weight of all other babies who had been born. (All this fuss about the scale was indoctrinated into your psyche long before you were even conscious of what a Size 8 *was*.) Since then, every time you visit your physician, you are weighed, and, again, compared to a set of averages.

Therefore, *ideal weight*, is a number based on a collection of averages. Medical professionals have used this number as one indicator for health. Those weighing forty percent or more over ideal body weight are labeled "clinically obese." And weighing 100%, or more, over ideal body weight is classified as "morbid obesity" which means weight is a separate and individual risk factor for dying.

One of the formulas for figuring "ideal" weight looks like this: For women, figure 100 pounds for the first five feet in height, and then five pounds for each additional inch. From this point, calculate 10% in either direction. For example, a woman who stands 5'5", would figure 100 pounds for the first five feet, then 25 additional pounds for the next five inches. From 125 pounds, she can go 12.5 pounds in either direction.

What's Healthy?

But let's get real. This formula may work for some depending on bone structure, lean body tissue, and a host of other parameters. But, we are not Barbie dolls, cracked out of a mold. We are human beings, who come in all sizes, shapes, and proportions. Let's stop calling it "ideal" weight, which can create a perfect setup for failure. Even the phrase, "goal" weight, implies something in the future that we vie after, but usually never attain. Why not ask yourself honestly, "what is my healthy, comfortable weight?" If you are 5'5" and haven't weighed 125 pounds since eight grade, that may be a clue it is not appropriate for you. On the other hand, if, at 5'5", weighing 235 pounds feels comfortable, it's time to be more honest with yourself. A "healthy" weight is one that will reduce life-threatening risk factors. And a "comfortable" weight is one you can maintain without constant struggle. Using your best judgment, choose a weight that is both healthy and comfortable for you. If you wish to, consult your physician.

Metabolic Factor

From you healthy, comfortable weight, you can calculate the next number that counts - your metabolic factor. Metabolism is the rate at which the body utilizes energy, or, more simply put, the number of calories the body *burns*. Metabolic **factor** is the number of calories *per pound* that the body burns just by existing. That means before any physical activity. According to numerous metabolic studies,[1] physically active women burn roughly 12 calories per pound, while sedentary women burn an average of 10 calories per pound. The difference is due to the fact that physically active people usually have a greater percentage of muscle versus fat than sedentary people do. And as you may already know, muscle is more metabolically active than fat, meaning that muscle burns more calories than fat. For purposes of averages, a metabolic factor of 11 is used in this book.

Each individual is different, therefore use your own judgment to determine which factor is appropriate for you. Nevertheless, don't be so quick to blame your weight on metabolism. Studies indicate that less than 3% of the overweight population has metabolic dysfunctions. On the other hand, if you have been sedentary for many years, your metabolic factor could drop as low as nine. What *does* impact metabolic rate? An exercise program that includes aerobics and weight training.

Average Daily Maintenance Calories

The next important number you want to know about is your average daily maintenance calories. These are the number of calories it takes to *maintain* a specific weight. Determine this number by multiplying your healthy, comfortable weight by your metabolic factor.

For example, the average daily maintenance calories of a 150-pound woman, before exercise, (using a metabolic factor of 11) are 1650. By exercising, she will burn additional calories depending on what she does. Let's say this hypothetical woman burns an additional 250 calories a day by walking. (You will learn more about calculating exercise calories in Chapter Three). This means she can eat an average of 1900 calories a day without gaining any weight. If she consistently eats more than that, she will store fat and gain weight. Obviously, no one eats exactly the same amount of calories every day, which is why we call them "average" maintenance calories. By looking at a week's worth of food calories for this 150-pound woman, you can see how her calories vary, but ultimately strike a balance at the 1900 mark.

DAY	TOTAL CALORIES	WHAT HAPPENED
Mon.	1775	A work day; She eats three light meals, including a mid-morning snack.
Tues.	1525	Her usual breakfast and lunch. She works late, skips dinner and stops for ice cream on the way home.
Wed.	2100	She goes out for dinner, has wine & dessert.
Thurs.	1850	Another day of eating three balanced meals, snacked on popcorn.

Fri.	2550	Goes out for Mexican food, including chips and margaritas.
Sat.	1720	Slept in, skipped breakfast, helped a friend move, grabbed a sandwich for lunch and a salad for dinner.
Sun.	1680	Went out for brunch, then ate a light dinner.

Her total calories for the week add up to 13,200. Divide this number by seven to get an average of 1885 calories a day. Now, suppose this 150-pound woman stopped at a fast food restaurant and ate a large cheeseburger, fries and a coke. This one meal supplies roughly 1400 calories, over 2/3 of her maintenance calories for the day. (More about food calories in Chapter Five.) By knowing her average daily maintenance calories, this woman now understands how this meal impacts her health and fitness. Take a moment to figure your average daily maintenance calories.

Can't Hurry Weight Loss

Have you ever seen something like this in a magazine, newspaper, or on TV?

"Lose 10 pounds in ONE WEEK!"

"Drop Five Pounds in Five Days Without Being Hungry!"

Not only have you seen it, you may have believed it. Or worse yet, tried it. The fantasy of losing weight quickly has been heavily fueled by the advertisements and weight loss scams to which you've been constantly exposed. Perhaps you *did* lose weight on those empty promises. But, did it stay off? Probably not. And most likely the weight you lost was water, not fat.

Is it even *possible* to lose 10 pounds in one week? Let's find out. First, you need to know that 3500 calories equals one pound of fat. Therefore, a ten-pound loss would mean a **35,000** calorie reduction (3500 x 10). And to deficit 35,000 calories in *one week* you'd have to reduce your food calories by 5000 a day! (35,000 ÷ 7 days) This is virtually impossible, unless you weigh over 500 pounds. The daily maintenance calories for a 500-pound woman are roughly 5500. Even in this case, the scenario is not a likely one.

Many experts recommend losing half a pound per week. Others feel one pound a week is OK. Even though this may sound excruciatingly slow, this is the kind of fat loss that stays off. Let's take Jane, whom you met in Chapter One, as an example. If Jane wanted to lose **one** pound of fat per week, she would need to deficit 3500 calories per week or 500 calories a day. If we subtract 500 calories from her 2200 maintenance calories (before exercise), she is left with 1700 food calories per day. This is do-able.

My Own Experience

When my second child turned six months old, I still needed to lose 25 pounds. Society gives women a built-in excuse for being overweight after childbirth, but that only lasts for a few months. To lose my excess weight I made a plan based on numbers. At 155 pounds, I burned 1700 calories a day. I expended an additional 250 calories doing physical activity, bringing my total calories burned to 1950. By decreasing my food calories to an average of 1700 per day, I was deficiting 250 a day or 1700 per week. This results in half a pound of fat per week. I followed the nutritional recommendations outlined in Chapter Four and kept an account of my food intake, Chapter Six. Sometimes the number on the scale wouldn't budge for days and I would feel discouraged. However, I didn't give up. I knew that for every 3500 calories I deficited, I was losing one pound of fat. (Even when the scale didn't say so.) The weight finally did come off, and it has stayed off.

3 Exercise: What, When, Why, and How Much

(Check with your physician before you begin any physical activity program.)

Everyone knows that exercise is good for you, right? We commonly see fit people riding bicycles in their brightly colored garb, running in their spandex, or sweating on stair machines.   However, studies indicate that those you see exercising are the minority of our population. According to government statistics,[1] since 1900, Americans have <u>decreased their physical activity by 75%</u>.
   In the early 1900's, a 125-pound woman consumed between 2000-2200 calories a day. Today, if a woman eats that many calories, she will weigh somewhere between 180 and 200 pounds. That is, *unless* she exercises. A woman who lived before our modern age, expended 300-500 calories a day participating in daily chores. Consider the activities of an early 1900's woman versus those of today's woman:

> *A woman who lived 100 years ago woke up in the*
> *morning to a cold home. To warm the house, cook*
> *meals and bathe, she had to build a fire. She walked*
> *to the barn for eggs, churned the butter and rolled*
> *out dough for bread. Back then, there were no*
> *Maytags, motor cars or push button ovens.*

A modern day female wakes up to take a hot shower, dress, and step into her car. She stops for coffee and a donut on her way to work. Sits at her desk in an office for eight hours. At five o'clock she drives home, pulls a frozen dinner out of the freezer, nukes it and eats.

Blame it on technology, from the automobile, right up to the microwave. We can't reverse technology, nor would most of us want to, yet the issue remains: A lack of exercise results in an unfit, unhealthy population.

Exercise And Cardiovascular Disease

Compared to *any* other lifestyle change, exercise is known to have the greatest impact on cardiovascular health. Studies indicate that by walking three to four hours per week, (approximately 30 minutes of walking per day) Americans can reduce their risk of heart disease by 60%. If walking sounds unappealing, consider how it might compare to having bypass surgery.

Exercise and Blood Lipids

At one time, blood cholesterol was the primary measurement for predicting the occurrence of atherosclerosis, the disease in which plaque clogs the arteries. We now know that cholesterol is only one part of an even more important number - the HDL ratio. HDL, which stands for "high density lipoprotein," is one of several fatty substances found in the blood stream. This one, called the "good" cholesterol, acts as a scavenger to remove the harmful blood cholesterols, called low density lipoproteins and very low density lipoproteins.[2] The HDL carries the LDL and VLDL to the liver where it is excreted. Therefore, a high ratio of HDL to total cholesterol is desirable. Exercise is known to increase HDL.

Blood Pressure & Exercise

Hypertension, often called the "silent killer" because it produces no obvious symptoms, is a major cause of heart attack and stroke. It is estimated that approximately 50 million Americans have high blood pressure. The criteria for determining "normal" versus "high" blood pressure was developed by the World Health Organization in 1978. The upper number (systolic) measures the pressure during the heart's contraction. The lower number (diastolic) measures pressure during the heart's resting phase. Each number above normal represents a degree of complication associated with heart disease, stroke and kidney disease.

Normal Blood Pressure = $\dfrac{140 \text{ or less}}{90 \text{ or less}}$

Borderline Hypertension = $\dfrac{141\text{-}159}{91\text{-}94}$

Hypertension = $\dfrac{160+}{95+}$

In a study where men with high blood pressure expended 2000 calories of physical activity per week (approximately one hour of walking per day), their risk for heart disease was decreased by 50%. In another study of over twenty different non-Westernized, rural cultures, where the population is physically active, absolutely **no** hypertension was found. Other studies within the US indicate that exercise helps hypertensive patients lower, or in some cases, completely end their medicated dosage.

Osteoporosis & Exercise

Osteoporosis is a disorder which causes fragile, porous bones resulting in bone loss and breakage. Drug companies and food manufacturers have jumped on the band wagon to promote pills and products in claims of preventing this disease. Even some cereal and orange juice companies add supplemental calcium to their products. Unfortunately, supplements have shown very little improvement in increasing bone density. What has shown improvement is **weight-bearing exercise.** "Weight-bearing" means walking, running, hiking or any activity in which your legs support you in resistance against gravity. One study of Asian women, who regularly carried weighted packs uphill, revealed they had virtually **no** bone loss. Coincidentally, these same women were eating a diet consisting of *less* than 800 milligrams of calcium per day, the current US RDA.

Exercise & Adult-Onset Diabetes

It is now known that 78% of **all** adult-onset diabetes is a direct result of excessive weight. On top of this, those who have been 40% or more above ideal body weight for a minimum of ten years, have an 80% chance of getting adult-onset diabetes. What reduces excess weight? You guessed it: Exercise.

Lean Body Tissue

After the age of 25 our bodies begin to lose lean body tissue. Over time this causes our metabolic rate to decrease which means an increase in body fat. Exercise, especially weight training, increases lean body tissue and helps maintain a metabolism that burns calories more efficiently.

Eat More, Gain Less

You already know that exercise burns additional calories. Therefore, it can safely be said that by exercising, you can eat more and gain less. By walking two or three miles a day you burn an extra 200 or 300 calories. This may not sound like a lot, but over one week, that's an extra 1400 - 2100 calories. In one year's time that's the equivalent of 20 - 30 pounds of fat.

Longevity

Numerous studies indicate that exercise increases longevity. Most recently, a study of over 25,000 men, conducted by Steve Blair at Cooper Institute for Aerobics Research in Dallas, concluded that "thin" men who were sedentary were nearly **three times** more likely to die young than "fat" men who exercised. This is not a push to gain weight, but another indicator that exercise is more important than the number on the scale.

Have We Covered Everything?

Exercise enhances every system of the body. It aids digestion, increases lung capacity and improves circulation. It keeps skin healthy and young looking. It reduces stress and anxiety which can lead to depression. And, because exercise is thought to enhance the immune system, it would be safe to say that people who exercise get sick less often. Scientists also speculate that when people exercise regularly, they are less susceptible to certain carcinogens, lowering the chances of getting specific cancers. It doesn't take a genius to figure out that exercise improves the overall quality of life.

How Much Is Enough?

Now that you know the benefits of physical activity, your next question might be: How much do I need to do? I remember an old adage that went like this :

EXERCISE FIVE TIMES A WEEK;
IMPROVE FITNESS.

EXERCISE THREE TIMES A WEEK;
MAINTAIN FITNESS.

EXERCISE TWO TIMES A WEEK OR LESS;
LOSE FITNESS.

The only problem with this is what one person calls "exercise," another calls "rest." During the 1970's, we heard the "no pain, no gain" motto. Then in the 1980's, low-impact took the lead and walking became popular. Not long afterward studies defined *exactly* how much exercise was needed to impact health and fitness. One of the most extensive of these was the 20-year, Stanford University School of Medicine, Paffenbarger study which included 17,000 men (sorry, ladies). Results showed that expending a minimum of 2000 calories per week in physical activity increased longevity and decreased heart disease by 30%. Expending 2000 calories means walking, bicycling, dancing, swimming, or any other aerobic exercise for 45 to 60 minutes a day. Interestingly, those individuals who expended *more* than 3500 calories per week (over 500 per day) did not gain any additional risk-lowering benefits. In fact, they became more likely to injure themselves and decrease their immune system response.

More Opinions

Experts, like Dr. William Castelli of the Framingham Heart Study, state that expending 1500 calories per week, the equivalent of a 200-calorie expenditure per day, is enough to offer protection against heart disease. Kenneth Cooper, MD, President and founder of the Aerobics Center, and author of the *New Aerobics for Women*, recommends thirty to forty minutes of continuous exercise, (working up to a pulse rate of 60 - 80% of maximal heart rate[3]) three to four times per week. This translates into roughly a 1500-calorie per week expenditure. He also recommends ten to fifteen minutes of weight training and stretching three times a week.

Taking all this into account, women need to engage in an exercise program that expends an average of <u>1500 to 1800 calories per week</u>. This means 45 - 60 minutes five to six days a week. If doing an activity for one hour sounds too overwhelming, try breaking it down into one minute increments. Then ask yourself "can I do this for five minutes?" Once you have achieved five minutes, add another five. Keep doing this over a period of several weeks until you've achieved 45 - 60 minutes. Expending more than 1800 calories a day is your option. Expending less than 1500 decreases optimum fitness and health benefits.

Calculating Exercise

Translating physical activity into calories is the most straight forward method of calculation. The number of calories burned depends on the muscles used, the weight of the participant, and the duration and intensity of the activity. Generally, activities that engage muscles of the *lower* half of the body burn 300 - 400 calories per hour. These would include walking, bicycling, hiking, and dancing. Running burns more depending on the distance traveled.

Activities that engage *upper* body muscles, which are half the size of the lower body muscles, burn 150 - 200 calories an hour. Gardening or housework would fall into this category. See the illustration on page 26.

Activities, such as rowing, cross-country skiing, swimming or an aerobics class all engage **both** the upper and lower muscles. These activities burn between 450 and 800 calories per hour, depending on the intensity. See the exercise barometer on page 28. Remember, all these numbers are averages and not meant for "splitting hairs." Your goal is progress, not perfection.

PHYSICAL ACTIVITY CALORIES PER HOUR

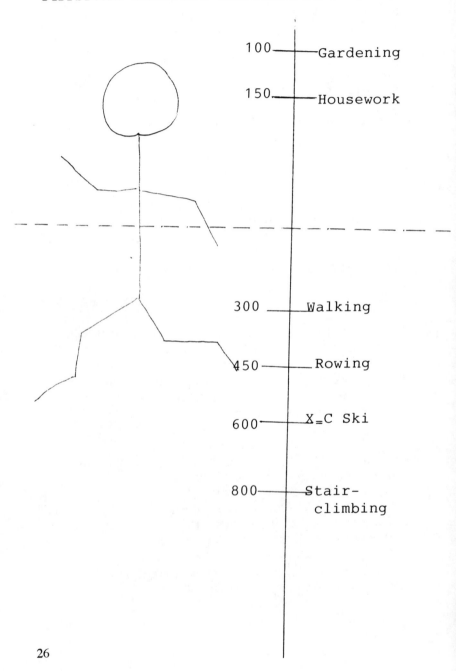

100 —— Gardening

150 —— Housework

300 —— Walking

450 —— Rowing

600 —— X=C Ski

800 —— Stair-
climbing

Size Counts

As mentioned earlier, body size affects calories expended. To illustrate this, imagine two boxes, one the size and weight of a refrigerator, another the size and weight of a toaster. Obviously, you would burn much more energy moving the larger box than you would moving the smaller one. Likewise a 300-pound person burns more calories walking a mile than does a 125-pound person.

To determine how much you burn, divide your weight by 150 (the standard) to get a weight factor. Then multiply this factor by the number of calories burned doing an activity. For example, for 200 pounds, divide 200 by 150 to get 1.3. Then, if you walk one mile, which burns 100 calories, multiply 1.3 times 100 to get 130 calories. For three miles, multiply 1.3 x 300 to get 390 calories. If you'd rather not use this calculation, refer to the following chart:

If you weigh...	For every mile, you burn....
130 pounds	85 calories
150	100
180	120
200	130
250	170
300	200

EXERCISE BAROMETER
(Based on 150-pound person per hour)[4]

ACTIVITY	CALORIES BURNED
Stairclimbing, running 8-10 mph. cross-country skiing,	800 - 1000
Walking uphill, running 4-6 mph, mountain biking, rowing	450 - 600
Walking 3-4 mph, bicycling 10 mph., rollerblading, alpine skiing	300 - 450
Walking 2-3 mph., heavy housework	200 - 300
Gardening, light house cleaning, strolling 1-2 mph.	100 - 200

Inclines Matter

For every mile you walk *uphill*, tack on an additional 50% more calories. For example, if you weigh 150 pounds, a three-mile walk on a **flat** surface burns 300 calories. Walking those same three miles at an incline adds another

150 calories, totaling 450. The same goes for bicycling mountain biking or cross-country skiing. For example ordinarily, a one-hour bike ride burns about 300 calories, but if you are biking uphill, this increases to a minimum of 450.

Barriers to Physical Activity

#1 "I'm too busy to exercise."

You're working full time, commuting an hour a day, and running a household. Who has *time* to exercise? It's true, few of us have time to squeeze another activity into our lives. Yet, to insure optimum health and fitness, exercise *must* be a priority. Can you commit thirty minutes of your day to a better quality of life? If your answer is "no," ask yourself this: How many times have I waited in line at the grocery store for 30 minutes? Or how often have I talked idly on the phone for 30 minutes? Or spent 30 minutes watching a mindless TV sitcom?

How can you creatively squeeze 30 minutes of exercise into your schedule? Is it possible to park half a mile away from your place of employment and walk? Can you join a gym and spend your lunch hour working out? Remember, every little bit counts. Park at the *farthest* space from the mall or grocery store. Take stairs instead of the elevator. Leave your car at home and walk whenever possible.

One client of mine who worked as a full time nurse and was raising four children on her own, barely had time to think, no less exercise. Only a unique solution would work for her to fit in 30 or 40 minutes of exercise five or six days a week. By probing into her daily routine I discovered a possible built-in plan for success. At the hospital where she worked, she took an elevator up ten flights of stairs five times a day. If she was willing to use the stairs instead, I calculated that she would expend 120 calories a day.[5] She agreed to give it a try. She arrived at work ten minutes early

29

to begin her climbing. At first she ascended slowly and cursed every step as sweat poured from her forehead. But, after a couple of weeks the climbing got easier. It wasn't long before she increased her caloric expenditure to 220 calories a day.

#2 "I'm not athletic"

A colleague of mine, now a successful weight consultant, began his fitness journey by walking to his mailbox and back *in the dark*. At the time, he weighed 420 pounds and was too ashamed to be seen exercising in public. After a few days, he increased his walk to halfway around the block. Then, all the way around. Slowly he began to lose fat and as his breathing became easier, he increased the distance to one mile. One of his biggest triumphs was walking two miles in the daylight. Eventually, he lost over two hundred pounds and now holds a world record for stair climbing. Before this, his prognosis was an early death. Now his risk factors have decreased and he lectures throughout the country. Before he walked out the door to his mailbox, he never considered himself "athletic."

Another client of mine was in a wheel chair, awaiting knee surgery, when I met her. Her physician would not operate until she lost 50 pounds. For her, exercise seemed out of the question, but we both worked hard to find a solution. Her arms, though weak, became our target. She started with 20 arm circles two times a day. Eventually she worked up to a total of 40 minutes of arm circles which burned about 100 calories. This not only improved her cardiovascular system, but also helped boost her morale. She finally had her surgery and is now walking to maintain her health and fitness.

#3 "It's raining, snowing, too dark or cold outside."

If you let the weather determine whether you get out of bed in the morning, you may find yourself under the covers all day. If you let the weather dictate your exercise habits, you may remain unhealthy and unfit for the rest of your life. Your job is to determine whether you need a rain slicker and boots, a coat and mittens, or a hat and sunscreen.

Obviously, it isn't wise to exercise in sub-zero degree weather or extreme heat. Otherwise, it is necessary to create alternatives. Take an aerobics class in a local gym. Buy a stationary bike for those cold, wintry nights. Or bundle up and walk through the snow! Join an indoor pool. Or jump rope. I once lived in a mountain town where it could snow for days without end. I was often held up inside. If I couldn't get out to walk or cross-country ski, I would turn on my favorite music and jump rope. Monotonous as it sounds, I was burning calories.

Beyond Aerobics

Stretching and weight training are also very important aspects of exercise. Daily stretching creates greater mobility and a sense of wellness. It brings more blood flow to the muscles and more oxygen and nutrients to the cells, promoting cell maintenance and repair. Elongating the muscles keeps them more supple and the skeletal system better aligned.

Ten to fifteen minutes of stretching per day can make a world of difference in how you feel. Remember, never strain your muscles. The key is to hold a gentle stretch for up to 30 seconds. Stretching at the end of your workout is as important as at the beginning. Bob Anderson's *Stretching* is an excellent resource. So is your community recreation department. Call to find out if the town offers any yoga or stretching classes.

Shaping Your Own Program

Now you are ready to begin your new exercise program. To create your own plan, choose an activity that satisfies your personal preference, fitness level, and time allotment. Remember, exercising is a lifetime commitment, so be sure to choose an activity that is fun for you. Exercise with a friend. Take a Nordic skiing or a folk dancing class. Don't hold back. If riding your bike sounds more like your style, start. If hiking up mountains thrills you, go for it!

Jane launched herself on a program, starting with 500 calories per *week*. She varied her choice of exercise between walking, stationary biking, and an aerobics class. Each day she posted the number of calories she burned on a calendar to measure her progress. Each week she added another 200 calories of exercise until she reached her goal of 1800. On the days she felt stiff and sore, she didn't give up. Most days she felt energized and strong.

If you have not exercised in quite some time, walking may be your preference. Begin slowly. You may start with as little as 300 calories per week. If so, walk one mile three times a week or half a mile six times a week. A half mile takes about 10 minutes. From this point, add more mileage every couple of weeks until you reach 1500 - 1800 calories per week. Whatever your choice of exercise, keep track of the number of calories you expend each day. This will give you perspective and encouragement. If you are in good enough condition to start at a higher level and increase at a more rapid rate, that's fine. Always consult with your doctor before starting a new exercise plan, especially if you have any medical problems.

In Summary

Remember, **not** doing physical activity creates a risk factor for disease. Keep track of your caloric expenditure to help motivate you to a goal of 1500-1800 per week. Every little bit counts. You deserve to be fit and healthy!

4 Nutrition: A Piece of Cake

Several years ago, my husband and I spent a weekend at a charming bed-and-breakfast house in the wine country of California. I was eight months pregnant, so wine tasting and hot-tubbing were off limits. Instead, we window-shopped and strolled (actually, I waddled) through the streets of the quaint vintage town.

The hallways of the B&B, which had at one time been a bordello, were lined with book-filled shelves. Many books had copyright dates as early as 1920. Scanning the titles, I found one dust-covered book printed in 1932 entitled, *Better Eating*. To my surprise, the recommendations read:

* Choose a variety of fresh fruits and vegetables.
* Eat an abundance of prepared whole grains and legumes.
* Choose proteins from chicken, fish and beef, avoiding fatty versions.
* Limit cooking with lard, and butter, as these contain fats.
* Eat dairy products sparingly.
* Drink 6-8 glasses of water a day.

Ironic, how we believe nutrition in our generation has taken a new age turn, when in fact, our grandparents probably practiced more natural wholesome eating than we can ever imagine. What has happened between then and now to create a nation of overweight, unhealthy individuals? One reason might be the over-abundance of processed and refined foods that we now consume. Born during the mid-1950's were "convenience" foods. As fast food restaurants claimed their fame for the most hamburgers sold, heart disease claimed a record number of lives.

Caveat Emptor

Today, facts about nutrition are abundant. All of us are barraged by statistics from the media, details on food containers, and unsolicited advice from relatives and friends. The problem is, that often, this information is contradictory, unreliable, or downright false.

Even the so-called "scientific" studies are confusing. One study claims that coffee raises blood pressure. Another insists that it's safe to drink up to five cups per day. One week you read that drinking red wine helps reduce cardiovascular disease. The next week you hear that alcohol increases your risk of cancer. How do you know what to believe? Just because it claims to be a "scientific" study doesn't mean you are given all the facts.

One particular study inferred that people who drink one or two glasses of beer or wine per day were shown to display a lower incidence of heart disease. Does this mean that beer and wine reduce the risk of heart disease? No.

What the study failed to take into account were **other** lifestyle-related factors of the people who drink only 1 or 2 glasses of beer or wine a day. The key issue in this study is moderation. Those who drink alcoholic beverages "moderately" are most likely moderate meat-eaters, fat-consumers, and exercisers. These last three behaviors contribute to lowering the risk for cardiovascular disease, not drinking beer or wine everyday. Once you've got the total picture, you can more accurately decide what to believe. If it sounds too good to be true, it probably is.

Several years ago, everything from ice cream to potato chips was advertised with claims of less fat, less salt, less of "whatever you believe isn't good for you." National food manufacturers came forth with the so-called "lite" foods and we, as consumers, ate it up.

At this same period, an olive oil manufacturer released its version of "light" oil. I was working in a medical facility at the time, counseling high-risk patients. During one of my lectures a woman announced that she had found a "lowfat" oil. When I tried to explain to her that oil, by its inherent nature, would never be "low" fat, she wouldn't believe me. The truth was, only the taste and color were lighter.

Other "light" foods such as chips, crackers, and cookies, all advertise "less oil." And they do have a tad less oil than the regular ones. But at 130 calories an ounce versus 150, eating five or six ounces will still get you in trouble. The bottom line is, sometimes, even the "lite" versions often contain too much fat. Fortunately, the government finally decided to regulate the use of the word "light. The bottom line: Don't rely on advertisements for your facts. Read labels and check for saturated fat.

"Fat-Free" items are another hot, yet in my opinion, controversial product. Don't rely on "fat-free" packaged foods to get your nutrients. Most of these are simple carbohydrates with an abundance of chemicals added. And even fat-free foods have calories.

An Apple a Day . . .

"Let me stress," says former Health and Human Services Secretary Louis Sullivan, "five servings a day (of fruit and vegetables) is minimum. If you can eat up to nine servings a day, all the better." Americans eat an average of 1.5 servings of fruit and vegetables per *week*. (And this includes the lettuce and tomato on burgers!) One serving of vegetables measures approximately half a cup. One serving of fruit weighs roughly five ounces.

Not only do fruit and vegetables supply essential vitamins, minerals, and fiber, they also help decrease the risk of diseases like diabetes, heart attack, stroke and cancer. All of these diseases together cause 70% of the deaths in our nation today.

The following headlines from news articles demonstrate the benefits of eating fruits and vegetables:

EAT YOUR CARROTS TO AVOID HEART ATTACKS, STROKES

DIET TIED TO BLADDER CANCER

ADD SALAD AND JUICE TO AVOID CANCER

MORE EVIDENCE FRUIT, VEGGIES FIGHT CANCER

BETA-CAROTENE: Nugget of Nutritional Gold

CRUCIFEROUS VEGETABLES CAN PREVENT CANCER

Excuses, Excuses, Excuses

Isn't it interesting how easily we construct excuses for not doing what we know will benefit us? Below I have listed the most common rationalizations for not eating fruit and vegetables.

Excuse # 1 *"Five servings a day? I could <u>never</u> eat that much food!"*

Those who believe "eating five or more servings of fruit and vegetables per day" is tantamount to gluttony are often the same people who think nothing of knocking off a bag of potato chips or half a dozen brownies. Half a pound of potato chips contain 1200 calories and half a dozen brownies easily supply 1500. On the other hand, an eight ounce baked potato or eight ounces of grapes check in at 160 calories. When you eat a minimum of five servings of fruit and vegetables per day, you are not as likely to reach for the chips or brownies.

Excuse # 2 *"Vegetables are too difficult and time-consuming to prepare."*

Is it really that difficult to peel a carrot, bake a potato or open up a can of green beans? The produce departments of most grocery stores now have pre-washed, pre-peeled and pre-cut veggies ready to eat or cook. If time is an issue, microwave or steam a large volume of potatoes, broccoli, squash, green beans or whatever vegetable you prefer and refrigerate them. Then during the week either reheat them or add them to a salad. Another time saver, if finances permit, is ordering steamed vegetables "to go" from your favorite restaurant. Avoid vegetables deep-fried or sautéed in butter or oil. Salad bars are another option. Just be sure to go easy on anything that contains mayonnaise or oil. Salad dressing at 80 calories per tablespoon needs taming also. Try using a fancy vinegar, or a low-oil dressing.

Excuse # 3 *"I don't like vegetables (or fruit.)"*

Maybe you don't like vegetables because your mother fed you overcooked Brussels sprouts when you were five years old. Now every time you think of a vegetable, you think of that distasteful experience. But, the truth is, there is more to the vegetable world than Brussels sprouts. (Besides, there are too many other reasons to blame our mothers.) We are all such creatures of habit, that sometimes we're not conditioned to try the new and unfamiliar. Many people get in a rut of eating only apples and bananas for their fruit. No wonder they are bored. If you like apples, try a different variety like Fuji or Braeburn. Did you know that there are over 300 varieties of vegetables at your local food market? Make a commitment to try one new fruit or vegetable each week. Make an exotic fruit salad with kiwis, mangoes, and papaya. Steam an artichoke, slice an avocado over your salad, or try arugula. If you really can't stand the sight of vegetables, you can always camouflage them in soups, casseroles, or stews.

Organic: It's Worth It!

Organic fruits and vegetables are those grown without chemical pesticides. Pesticides, like processed and refined foods, came along during the 1950's. Then touted as a miraculous discovery, these chemicals were sprayed indiscriminately upon massive harvests. Decades later, a possible link between pesticides and cancer has been discovered. Organically grown fruits and vegetables cost nearly twice that of commercially grown ones, but don't let that deter you. If you quit buying the outrageously-priced packaged snack foods, you'll have enough to purchase the organics. Besides supplying more nutrients, the organics taste like "real" food, not a plastic imitation. Shop at farmer's market, or visit your local health food store and see for yourself.

The Facts About Fat

Protein, carbohydrates, (alcohol) and fats all supply us with calories. When we classify each of these into units of "calories per gram", it becomes evident why eating too much fat can make you "fat."

Protein	=	4 calories per gram
Carbohydrate	=	4 calories per gram
Fat	=	9 calories per gram
Alcohol	=	7 calories per gram

(Alcohol is metabolized and stored similarly to fat)

Dietary fats are made up of carbon and hydrogen molecules. A "saturated" fat is fully hydrogenated, meaning there is no room for any more hydrogen atoms. Saturated fats, found in animal products, palm and coconut oil, increase the level of total cholesterol and LDL cholesterol. When these cholesterols are elevated, the formation of atherosclerotic plaque and the risk of cardiovascular disease increase.

Polyunsaturated fats have room for at least four more hydrogen molecules. These fats help <u>lower</u> total cholesterol and also provide linoleic acid, an essential fatty acid that our bodies need, yet can not produce on their own. Polyunsaturated fats are found in sunflower, safflower, sesame, corn and soybean oils. Although polyunsaturated fats have been recommended over saturated fats, it's important to know that these fats also reduce HDL cholesterol. If you recall, HDL cholesterol is the "good" cholesterol that scavenges the bad fat from the bloodstream.

Mono-unsaturated fats have *two* spaces left for hydrogen atoms to bond with the carbon atoms. These fats lower **both** total cholesterol <u>and</u> LDL cholesterol levels, yet do not lower the HDL. Therefore mono-unsaturated fats are the best choice for decreasing the risk of cardiovascular disease. Mono-unsaturated fats are found in olive oil, canola oil, peanut oil and avocados.

How Much Is Too Much?

You automatically get more than twice the amount of calories by eating fat than you would eating protein or carbohydrate. And, as you know, unused calories are stored as fat. An interesting and significant study published in the University of California Wellness Letter (October 1988) revealed how differently our bodies use and store calories derived from fat versus those from carbohydrates. During the study, when individuals ate 100 calories from carbohydrate, 23 of those were utilized in the process of metabolism, leaving only 77 to be expended or stored. When these same individuals ate 100 calories from fat, only 3 of those were used up in the metabolic process, leaving 97 calories to be stored.

It has been recommended by certain health institutions that Americans eat a diet that consists of no more than 30% fat. But other experts disagree, saying this is not low enough, and 10% is better for reducing health risks. A ten percent diet can be radical and even unrealistic. A diet consisting of 20-25% may be a more practical approach. To figure fat grams, multiply either .20 or .25 by your average daily maintenance calories. This gives you the number of calories of fat you can eat per day. Then divide this number by nine (nine calories per gram of fat). You now have the number of fat grams you can eat per day.

Still other authorities now say that it's the "saturated" fat that is the culprit, not the "total" fat. Yet, since most of the food choices that we Americans eat are saturated fats, you can't go wrong by decreasing all fats.

Yet, fat is certainly not *completely* bad. We do need fat in our diet to help transport fat-soluble vitamins to cells and regulate hormones. Fat supplies our bodies with a concentrated form of energy, and gives skin and hair a supple texture.

Fat Sources

Most of us are familiar with the obvious fats, such as oil, butter, margarine, mayonnaise, salad dressings, nut butters and visible fat found around the edges of meats like steak and pork chops. But don't forget the foods that combine fat with simple carbohydrates. These include pastries, cookies, crackers, donuts, cakes, and chips. Then, there are the foods that contain fat and protein or dairy products, like ice cream, cheese, red meats such as Prime rib, salami and pepperoni, dairy products such as sour cream, whipping cream, half & half and whole milk products.

Carbohydrates

Fresh baked bread with *butter,* potatoes pooled with *gravy,* and pasta soaked in a creamy *cheese* sauce are often the images that come to mind when you hear the word "carbohydrate." This is most likely how carbohydrates have inherited their notoriously wicked reputation. The fact is it's not the carbs that cause a dietary disaster - it's the saturated fat!

> One slice of bread contains one gram
> of fat.
> Butter contains 12 grams per tablespoon.
>
> Potatoes serve you ZERO grams of fat.
> It's the gravy that gets you.
>
> Pasta served in a tomato or wine-based sauce can
> taste just as yummy for 50% less fat calories than the
> cheesy ones.

Make it Simple to Eat Complex

In a society where the most advertised and readily available foods are simple carbohydrates laden with fat, eating complex carbohydrates can be a challenge. Simple carbohydrates contain one unit of sugar per molecule and consist of sugars, in the form of fruits, table sugar, molasses, honey or corn syrup. Complex carbohydrates, which supply energy for cell growth and maintenance, contain several units of sugar per molecule and consist of starches in their most natural form.

Simple: (sugars)
 * fruit
 * refined sugar: sucrose, fructose, maltose, dextrose
    foods that have had sugar added to them:
    cereals, candy, cookies, crackers

<u>Complex</u>: (starches)
  * vegetables
  * whole grains: oats, barley, wheat, rye, millet, corn, rice
  * whole grain breads, whole grain cereals & pastas legumes such as peas, lentils, kidney beans, white, black, Pinto and garbanzo. Legumes contain about 50% protein and 50% carbohydrate.

National health organizations advise eating a diet that consists of between 60-65% carbohydrate. For a 140-pound woman, this means eating approximately 1000 calories of carbohydrates per day with the majority of those being complex.

Unfortunately, if you are like most Americans you are getting a large percentage of your food calories from simple carbohydrates and fat. You don't normally find fresh fruit, steamed vegetables, brown rice, baked potatoes, black bean soups or whole grains as readily as you find fried rice, French fries, canned soup, potato chips, cookies, and white bread. The more processed a food, the less nutrients it contains.

Look at what happens to food when it has been processed:

NATURAL	PROCESSED
whole oats	**granola bar** (fiber removed, fat & sugar added)
apple	**apple juice** (fiber removed, sugar increased)
baked potato	**potato chips** (fat added, nutrients & fiber removed)
brown rice	**white rice** (fiber & nutrients removed)

corn (on cob)	cream corn (sugar, fat & salt added)
whole grain bread	**Wonder bread** (nutrients & fiber removed)

In most instances, processing removes fiber, water, minerals, and vitamins, especially B-complex. Vitamin B-complex assists in the functioning of the heart, muscles, and nervous system. It also helps keep skin, nails and hair healthy. A lack of this vitaman complex precipitates a host of health problems.

Not only are nutrients lost during refinement, but ingredients, such as salt, sugar, chemical preservatives and fat are *added*. And these are of what our bodies need less, not more. A general rule of thumb is to eat foods in their most natural form.

Fiber

Remember oat bran? About ten years ago it became evident that the fiber contained in the bran of oats significantly reduced blood cholesterol. To help you understand why, let's go back to a simple lecture on fiber.

There are two kinds of fiber: Insoluble and soluble. Insoluble fiber went through its own fashionable era starring wheat bran. "Insoluble" means not water soluble. Foods high in insoluble fiber travel through the intestinal tract at a more rapid pace. This is known to help reduce constipation, diverticulosis and possibly even colon cancer. Fifteen to twenty years ago people were buying bagfuls of wheat bran and adding it to juice, cereal and main dishes to reap the benefits.

The oat bran craze emerged from an effort to reduce cholesterol. Oat bran contains a high percentage of *soluble* fiber. This type of fiber helps reduce blood cholesterol by soaking up and excreting bile acids which contain

43

cholesterol. Food manufacturers packed oat bran, this previously "unheard of" substance, into every food possible. What was not advertised was that eating a diet of fresh fruits, vegetables, and whole grains would also supply a bona fide amount of both types of fiber and keep digestion and blood cholesterol in tiptop shape.

Sodium

Salt is another issue. According to many studies, unless you have hypertension (high blood pressure) or a kidney problem, (in which case you need to consult your physician) salt is not necessarily a major health risk. Yet, other studies indicate that in cultures where no salt is used, hypertension is virtually nonexistent.

Americans take in over 3000 milligrams of sodium a day. To decrease your risk of high blood pressure, it is advised you take in no more than one gram a day (1000 milligrams). Let this be a reminder the next time you reach for the salt shaker. Read the labels on canned and packaged foods for sodium levels. Notice the difference in the levels of sodium in these foods.

corn (fresh)	1 cup	=	trace
corn flakes	1 cup	=	320 mg
corn chips	15	=	300 mg.
corn (can)	1 cup	=	400 mg

3 oz. turkey roasted	=	100
1 baked potato	=	0
1//2 c. green beans	=	0
Total		100 mg.

1 Froz. Turkey Dinner	=	1,500
Total		1500 mg.

Protein: Have We Been Brainwashed?

In this Westernized culture of ours, few people need to worry about getting enough protein. In fact, the opposite is more often the case. Why do we believe we need to eat an abundance of protein? Perhaps we've been brainwashed by the powerful beef lobbyists and their tremendous advertising budget. Or maybe the scarcity of meat during the depression caused the notion that this food was a luxury, as well as a sign of better economic times. Whatever the reason, our thinking must shift.

According to the World Health Organization, the Food and Nutrition Board and the National Research Council our daily needs for protein range between two and a half to eight percent of our total caloric intake. (Protein requirements change during growth, pregnancy and lactation.) The average American consumes a forty percent protein diet. Too much protein causes stress on the kidneys, and inhibits the absorption of certain minerals, especially calcium. And since most protein choices are derived from animal sources, high in saturated fat, the result is an increased risk of cardiovascular disease and cancer. Reducing protein to 15% of your total caloric intake will supply you with enough, but not too much.

Choosing protein that comes from plant, rather than animal sources can help reduce saturated fats and risk factors. Combinations of legumes, grains, and vegetables all furnish the essential amino-acids our bodies need. Purchase a vegetarian cookbook and try one recipe per week. You may discover that you like meatless meals.

Calcium

Calcium, one of the many important minerals we need in our diets, has in the last decade attracted ample press.   In addition to keeping bones strong and healthy, calcium helps regulate the heart, muscles, and nerves. Without enough calcium in your diet, your body draws calcium from it's own reserves - your skeletal system. This leaves bones depleted, frail and at an increased risk for osteoporosis. Osteoporosis, which usually occurs with aging, is a disease that causes thinning and weakening of the bones.

In this society, with the indoctrination of the National Dairy Council, milk products are esteemed as the superior source of calcium. The National Institute of Health's latest recommendation for women who want to prevent osteoporosis is 1000-1200 milligrams of calcium per day. To achieve this goal, we turn to more dairy products. Although, it is true that dairy products contain high levels of calcium, they also contain a high content of protein which has been shown to *inhibit the absorption* of calcium. Studies indicate that in cultures where there is little protein consumption and even less dairy, there is also little or no incidence of osteoporosis. Few people realize that vegetables are an excellent source of calcium. One cup of collard greens contains 300 milligrams of calcium, as does a cup of milk. The difference is that vegetables also contain a calcium-absorbing mineral called boron. Try to include as many vegetables as you can in your daily diet.

Milligrams of calcium in vegetables:

Kale, 1 cup	200
Mustard greens, 1 cup	190
Spinach, 1 cup	165
Broccoli, 1 cup	135
Bok choy, 1 cup	115
Swiss Chard	105

Vitamin Supplements

Due to the depletion of the earth's soil, the toxins in the air and water, and the amount of stress in our lives, taking a good multi-vitamin/anti-oxidant supplement is highly recommended. Yet, this should never be a substitute for eating wholesome, natural foods.

In Summary

Use the recommendations mentioned in this chapter to design your food plan. Eat a minimum of five servings of fruits and vegetables per day, organic if possible. Remember to eat foods in their most natural form. Limit processed and refined foods. Complex is better than simple in the carbohydrate department. Remember to choose a variety of foods to avoid toxicity. When eating fats, choose mono-unsaturated over saturated. To further your knowledge of nutrition check the multitude of health and nutrition books at your local bookstore.

When you are ready, go on to the next chapter. If you find that you are eager to read about the emotional component of overeating, skip ahead to Chapter Seven, and come back to the calorie chapter later.

5 Calories: The Good, the Bad, and the Ugly

The first thing people say when calories are mentioned, is, *"It's fat that counts, not calories."* Ah! But this chapter will enlighten you. The fact is, it is nearly impossible **not** to speak of calories when referring to health and fitness.

* When nutrition is mentioned, calories are mentioned. Calories are the basis from which the percentage of fat, carbohydrate, and protein is calculated.

* Calories translate the rate of metabolism. Women burn 11 calories per pound. Men burn 12 calories per pound.

* To lose one pound of fat, one needs to deficit 3500 calories. Fat contains nine calories per gram. Protein and carbohydrates contain four calories per gram.

* Calories offer a sound method for calculating physical activity and a tangible measure for setting goals. Walking two miles a day burns approximately 200 calories, which over one year keeps off twenty pounds of fat.

Calories Kept in Context

One of the reasons calories have received such a bad rap is that they have been taken completely out of context. For example, knowing that an eight-ounce steak contains 800 calories may mean very little to you. But if you weigh 140 pounds, and know that this steak absorbs over half of your daily caloric allotment, 800 calories suddenly takes on a new meaning.

Suppose while dining out at her favorite restaurant, Jane ordered grilled halibut instead of her usual NY steak. If both orders contained eight ounces, the steak, at 100 calories per ounce, yields 800 calories, whereas the halibut, at 30 per ounce, supplies 240. With a savings of 560 calories Jane could still enjoy the following foods:

salad w/2T dressing	170 calories
5 ounce baked potato	100
w/ 1 T sour cream	30
6 ounces white wine	120
2 ounces French bread	150

Compare the caloric difference of the two sandwiches below:

Roast Beef Sandwich		vs.	Turkey Sandwich	
4 oz. roast beef	400		4 oz. turkey	200
2 sl. bread	200		2 sl. bread	200
2 T mayo	200		2 T. mustard	60
lettuce/tomato	10		lettuce/tomato	10
	810			470

If this 340-calorie difference doesn't impress you, think again. Choosing the turkey with mustard, instead of the roast beef with mayonnaise, four times a week would reduce one's body fat by **twenty** pounds over one year's time.

This doesn't mean you have to eat halibut and turkey sandwiches with mustard everyday for the rest of your life. What it does illustrate is that making changes based on calorie knowledge significantly impacts body fat and health. In other words, calories **do** count!

Of course, *knowing* calories doesn't mean you will always choose the appropriate foods. (Especially if you are eating for unresolved emotional reasons, discussed in Chapter Seven.) On the other hand, realizing the consequences of certain food selections, offers a greater opportunity for empowering you. Don't remain a victim of random consequences by ignoring calories.

What is a calorie?

Like most people, you probably learned the definition of a calorie in your high school science class. And, chances are, you don't remember that a calorie is the *amount of energy it takes to raise the temperature of one gram of water one degree centigrade.* Calories are derived from protein, carbohydrates, and fat. All which nourish our bodies. Alcohol, another source from which we gain calories, renders no nutritional value. (Although the beer companies would love to make us think so). Water, fiber, vitamins and minerals which are all essential to our health and well-being, do not contain calories.

A Delicate Balance

For our bodies to perform their functions, we need a certain number of calories. The amount of energy we "deposit" in our bodies (food) versus the amount we "expend" (bodily functions and exercise) creates a balance we define as either fit or fat. If we take in more calories than we burn, our bodies act like little pack rats storing this excess energy as fat. Every 3500 calories we store produces one pound of fat. To lose fat, we need to reduce the amount of calories we take in, either through food calorie reduction, exercise or both. The problem is, most people believe they must starve to be fit. Not so!

I remember meeting a friend for lunch one day who was always trying to lose weight. I never give unsolicited advice, so I bit my tongue when she ordered,

> *a Caesar salad,*
> *a tiny plate of pate and cheese,*
> *and a few slices of fruit.*

I ordered,

a plate of linguini with red sauce,
a dinner salad with lowfat dressing
and a glass of wine.

I munched on French bread (no butter, of course) as we waited for our orders to arrive. She drank several glasses of water. Once our food came I noticed her watching as I finished my generous portion of noodles. "I don't understand how you can eat so much without gaining weight," she remarked. If she had been knowledgeable about calories, she'd have known that her lunch stacked up close to 1000, while mine was only 400.

The Barometer System

To calculate food calories, you need a system. The system utilized in this book is based on a sliding scale of averages translated into calories *per weight ounce.*[1]

Each <u>similar</u> type of food is assigned a number representing an average. These numbers are placed on a barometer beginning at zero calories per ounce and ending at 250 per ounce. **All** foods are included within this range. The system works this way. Take cake as an example: Angel food cake, the lowest calorie cake which contains no fat, supplies 100 calories per ounce. Carrot cake,[2] on the other hand, which contains a lot of oil, supplies the highest number of calories at 140 per ounce. Therefore, to assess the calories of cake, we come up with an average of 120 per ounce. So, the next time you are eating a piece of double chocolate fudge cake that tastes like a 2000 calories, you can be assured that it contains 120 per ounce. The next, and equally crucial, step is to know how much your piece of cake weighs. A piece of cake can weigh anywhere in the vicinity of three to ten ounces. Figure that out.

By memorizing a handful of numbers, you will eventually be able to calculate the calories of nearly any food that exists. The more you use it, the better you get. At first this system may seem foreign to you, but the more you refer to it, the more simple it becomes. A blank worksheet appears on page 56. Fill it in as you read through the chapter. A completed barometer appears at the end of this chapter.

Why Not Use a Calorie Book?

You may be wondering why you should learn calories according to "weight ounce" when you can look them up in a book? Suppose for a moment, that every morning you eat a muffin for breakfast. This is what happens when you rely on a calorie book:[3]

Muffin, blueberry,...............116 cal.

Blueberry ,small...................125

Bran, medium.....................106

Corn, medium.......................106

Bran, 2" diameter....................156

Calorie counting books describe muffins in either diameter inches or as small, medium and large. Both of these methods of description are confusing and inaccurate. Taking the books as truth, let's say you appraise *your* muffin at 125 calories.

Now, let's turn to the barometer system. Muffins, as you will learn later, supply 100 calories per ounce (unless they are prepared without fat; recipe on page 99) and can weigh anywhere from three to eight ounces. This means they supply between 300 and 800 calories. Let's say your muffin is an average sized one that weighs four and a half ounces. Now, think of the consequences of eating a 450 calorie muffin and believing it is 125 calories. Over a year's time those additional 325 calories will add 34 pounds of fat on your body that you cannot explain, because you believed the calorie books.

Let me stress, that I am not "condemning" the foods that are located at the high end of the barometer, but rather calling your attention to the fact that eating an abundance of these foods will probably put you over your average daily maintenance calories, which means gaining fat.

Starting at the top: Oils

Obviously, the more fat a food contains, the more calories it contains. Therefore oils, which consist of 100% fat, top the barometer at 250 calories per ounce. (125 calories per tablespoon) This includes all oils, regardless of whether they are mono-unsaturated, polyunsaturated, or saturated. Foods that *contain* oil will also be higher on the barometer than those that do not. For example, French fries, which are cooked in oil, supply 100 calories per ounce, while baked potatoes supply 20 per ounce.

What about butter?

Since butter is 100% fat, wouldn't it yield 250 calories per ounce, as does oil? No, because butter contains up to 15% water. And since water contains zero calories, it brings the calories of butter down to 200 per ounce. (100 calories per tablespoon.)

Perhaps you stopped using butter because it is a saturated fats which increases the risk of heart disease. Instead, you use margarine, a polyunsaturated fat, to help reduce that risk. Yet, recent studies also link hydrogenated oils, found in margarine, to high blood cholesterol levels. When margarine, originally an oil, is changed into a solid form, by a process called hydrogenation, the molecules become similar to those of saturated fats. Does this mean you should go back to eating butter? Not necessarily. These studies are not meant to promote a return to the use of butter. Instead, they render more data about the fact that we can **not** readily substitute one fat for another. Margarine contains 200 calories per ounce too, unless it is the lowfat version.

So what do you do? Skip the butter or margarine altogether and spread jam on your toast and low fat sour cream on your baked potatoes. Cooking with a little olive oil is fine, but don't forget to experiment with herbs, wine, (the alcohol cooks out) and different spices whenever you can.

Peanut Butter and Mayonnaise

Peanut butter and mayonnaise also fall at 200 calories per ounce (100 calories per tablespoon). If you are accustomed to lathering mayonnaise on your sandwiches, think of how much you might enjoy a spicy mustard at 15 calories a tablespoon instead. If you dislike mustards try one of the "light" versions of mayonnaise at only 50 calories per tablespoon. Peanut butter, a polyunsaturated fat, can be used as a protein source. Just use it frugally, since it is 80% fat.

The Anchor

From oils at the very top, slide down to the bottom of the barometer at zero. Water, so necessary for our survival, and a component of so many foods, serves as the perfect anchor for the barometer. Just as foods with a high percentage of fat contain more calories, foods with a large percentage of water contain less. For example, most fruits and vegetables, contain under 20 calories per ounce. Watermelon, because of its high content of water, contains only eight.

Adding water to foods during cooking also decreases the calories proportionately. For example, uncooked rice, at 110 calories per ounce, drops to 30 calories per ounce once

THE CALORIE BAROMETER

Calories Per Ounce

250
200
175
150
120
110
100
75
50
25
20
15
10
5
0

it has been cooked and the water has been absorbed. (More on grains later in this chapter.) As the water content in foods decrease, the number of calories increases. For example, dried fruit climbs up the barometer because the water has been removed. Peaches, apricots and apples, normally 15 calories per ounce, move up to 70 per ounce once they have been dried. Grapes, which supply 20 calories per ounce, shoot up to 90 as raisins.

Fruit and Vegetables

Packed with vitamins and minerals, fruit and vegetables taste great, and supply the least number of calories of any other foods. Leafy and watery vegetables like celery, lettuce, radishes, mushrooms, and peppers start at three calories per ounce. The stalkier ones like zucchini and green beans get five calories per ounce. As sugar and starch content increases, so do calories. For example, carrots, broccoli, cabbage, and cauliflower average 10 calories per ounce, while potatoes and corn go up to 20 per ounce. None of these contain more than 0.2 grams of fat.

Fruits start a bit higher than vegetables on the caloric barometer, because of their natural sugar content. Lemons are lowest at five calories per ounce. Melons are next at ten. Most others fall between 12 and 16 calories per ounce. A simple rule of thumb is to give all fruits 15 calories per ounce, except for grapes at 20 and bananas at 25. Avocados, the exception to the rule, contain 50 calories per ounce due to their high fat content.

If you are in doubt about the calorie content of a certain vegetable, just ask yourself "what does it most resemble?" For example, a potato supplies 20 calories an ounce, so how many calories would you give a sweet potato? A sweet potato contains more sugar than a regular potato, therefore tagging it a tad higher would make sense. Sweet potatoes contain 25 calories per ounce. What about asparagus? Asparagus, a stalky vegetable resembles broccoli in texture, so if you guessed 10 calories per ounce, you're catching on. Remember, any vegetable that has been deep fried or marinated in oil will jump to 100 calories per ounce.

This is how fruits and vegetables look on the barometer:

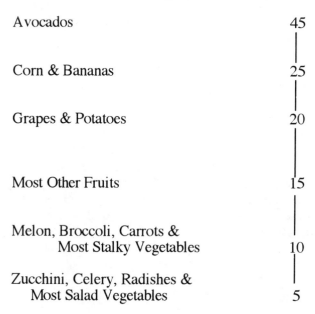

Avocados	45
Corn & Bananas	25
Grapes & Potatoes	20
Most Other Fruits	15
Melon, Broccoli, Carrots & Most Stalky Vegetables	10
Zucchini, Celery, Radishes & Most Salad Vegetables	5

Smack, Crackle, Pop: Dry Carbohydrates

Dry cereal, flour, sugar, uncooked pasta, rice, and grains are all classified as "dry" carbohydrates. These contain neither fat nor water and are located smack in the middle of the barometer at 110 calories per ounce.

Once cooked, pasta and rice drop down to around 30 per ounce due to water absorption. The most accurate method for calculating pasta and rice calories is to weigh them dry, *then* cook them. For example, two ounces of dry pasta supplies 220 calories. Once it's cooked, it yields roughly one and a half cups. Rice is smaller than pasta and packs more into a cup. Two ounces of uncooked rice at 220 calories yield a little over a cup. The next time you eat cold cereal notice the nutritional information on the package. Even the sugary cereals like Frosted Flakes® and Trix® supply 110 calories per ounce because sugar is a dry carbohydrate too. If a cereal provides more than 110, that's a clue it contains fat, usually in the form of nuts or oil. i.e. granola. Each ounce of cereal yields approximately 2/3 cup to 3/4 cup. A dense cereal, like Grapenuts®, supplies 1/4 cup per one ounce, while the airy ones, like Kix® or puffed rice, will yield one to one and a quarter cups per ounce.

Bread

If flour provides 110 calories per ounce, then wouldn't bread be the same? Bread is not a "dry" carbohydrate since it contains water. Bread supplies an average of 75 calories per ounce. Those that contain fat go as high as 90.

Muffins, similar to bread in texture, contain sugar and fat which moves them higher up on the barometer to 100 calories per ounce. Unfrosted cake also contains 100 calories per ounce. Once frosted, it jumps to 120.

Chocolate

I've heard some women say they'd rather curl up on the couch with a box of chocolates than with a man. Sometimes, I don't exactly blame them, but, when it comes to fitness or health, you might be better off with the man. Chocolate, made up of sugar (110 calories per ounce) and cocoa butter (200 calories per ounce), lands at 150 per ounce. An average candy bar weighs close to two ounces totaling 300 calories. This is not a recommendation to completely deprive yourself of chocolate. A little bit once in a while can't hurt. On the other hand, if one piece leads to half a dozen, you may be better off choosing something else.

Sometimes the sugar we crave can be satisfied by eating fruit. Try it sometime, you might be surprised by the results.

Bet You Can't Eat Just One

The advertisement was right, no one ever eats only "one potato chip." At 150 calories per ounce, a bag of potato chips can be a perfect way to self-destruct. If you're wondering what potato chips do to your fat cells, think about how slimy your fingers feel after you've been dipping into them. Next time you're in the mood to munch - try pretzels, raw vegetables or air-popped popcorn instead. If you can not forgo butter on your popcorn, try a mixture of 1/2 tablespoon melted butter and 1/2 tablespoon water. Six cups of popcorn, including the butter, will supply 200 calories, three grams of fiber and five grams of fat (from the butter). A cup and a half of chips supplies 450 calories, no fiber and 30 grams of fat.

Other Snacks

Most snack foods contain a combination of flour, sugar and fat. The result: an average caloric content of 120 per ounce. Those that contain no fat, like saltines, Rye-Krisp® or rice cakes, contain 110 per ounce. The next time you're at the grocery store, read the labels on the cracker boxes. Try to avoid those containing hydrogenated oils. Cookies, cakes, pastries and donuts also fall at this 120 calorie-per-ounce point. A great solution for not eating high-fat snacks is **not buying them**! Stock your pantry, refrigerator, and cupboards with fresh fruits, vegetables, pretzels, rice cakes or no-fat cookies. (Recipe for cookies on page 108.)

Nuts To You

The next time you grab a handful of cashews at a cocktail party or you're munching on peanuts in front of the TV, remember, nuts contain a whopping 170-180 calories per ounce, 600 to 800 calories per cup and an average of 75 - 80% fat. Seeds, rich in Vitamin E, contain roughly 160 per ounce. Eat these sparingly.

Fish, Meats, and Poultry

The calories of red meat, fish and poultry are determined by their raw weight. Animal protein shrinks after it's been cooked, losing mostly water. Therefore according to the US Department of Agriculture, the raw-weight method is the most accurate. A raw eight-ounce steak can shrink to six ounces once it's been cooked. Yet, it will still contain 800 calories.

Where's the Beef?

There are so many claims about the "lean-ness" of red meat, that it's no wonder people are confused. The meats with the highest content of fat - prime rib, sausage, salami and pastrami, contain the highest calories - 120 per ounce. The leanest cuts of beef, lamb and pork (with all visible fat cut off) supply 90 calories per ounce. All the rest are 100 calories per ounce.

One client of mine, I'll call Diane, was determined that no matter what she had to give up eating, it would not be beef. Diane believed that beef was the best choice of protein she could serve her family of four growing boys. Dinner consisted of beef, pork or lamb five nights a week. Another night she dined at her favorite prime rib restaurant and the remaining evening was pizza. It was no wonder she had a weight problem. My job was to convince her that making choices like fish, chicken and legumes would help her and her family maintain better health.

Diane's first assignment was to dine at a seafood restaurant. I explained how she could cut calories and fat in half by choosing poached salmon, steamed lobster, grilled swordfish, baked Mahi Mahi, or Teriyaki halibut instead of beef. Each week she had an excuse for not going. The only fish she remembered eating were frozen fish sticks on Friday nights. Finally, after three weeks, she reluctantly dragged herself to a fish restaurant. That night, she phoned me to report how "meaty" and "delicious" swordfish was. Each week she went back to the restaurant to try a new selection of fish.

Diane's next assignment was to prepare chicken one night a week. She was pleasantly surprised with recipes from a lowfat cooking magazine. Finally, she decided fish and poultry were choices she could live with, but still refused to try a legume. Only when I prepared a lentil stew (recipe on page 103) and brought it to our session did she sample a taste. Amazingly, she liked it. She promised to try another bean recipe and add that to her repertoire of dinners. With these food changes, leaving one night per week for red meat, she decreased her caloric intake by 500 calories a day, which helped reduce her weight by 45 pounds.

More and more people are substituting fish, poultry and vegetarian choices for red meat. Try a recipe in one of the many vegetarian cookbooks now available. Learn more about the liabilities of eating red meats by reading *Diet For a New America*, by John Robbins.

Poultry

Chicken, turkey, and Cornish hen range from 40 calories per ounce for white breast meat without the skin to 65 per ounce for dark meat with the skin. To keep it simple, give all poultry 50 calories per ounce, except duck. Duck, abundant in fat for purposes of buoyancy and insulation contains 125 calories per ounce. Baking, broiling or poaching poultry maintains 50 calories per ounce. Cooking with fat causes calories to climb. Deep-fried chicken goes up to 125 per ounce.

Eggs contain 45 calories per ounce. An average egg weighs two ounces. Poached or boiled maintains the calories at 45, while scrambling in butter or oil moves that up. A four-egg omelet with cheese cooked in butter can whip up over 600 calories. The current recommendation for consumption of eggs is four per week.

Fish

Fish ranges between 25 and 50 calories per ounce. Shellfish, (shrimp, lobster & crab) and white fish contain 25 calories per ounce. Salmon, mackerel, and sardines, high in omega-3 fatty acids, help reduce cholesterol and contain 50 calories per ounce. Tuna packed in water supplies 30 per ounce. (Double that for the oil-packed version.)

Cheese

One ounce of cheese contains an average of 100 calories with nearly 80% of those from fat. Cheddar is highest on the list, mozzarella the lowest. Cottage cheese supplies 80 to 120 calories per half cup depending on the fat content. Use cheese as a flavor-enhancer grated over vegetables, soups and pastas. One *grated* ounce goes a long way. On crackers, try a lowfat version, but limit the quantity.

Pizza

Speaking of cheese, what about pizza? Pizza consists of bread, cheese, tomato sauce, veggies or meat. Bread supplies 75 calories per ounce and cheese 100, so without much further calculation you could estimate pizza at 90. Pepperoni or sausage toppings increase calories to 100 per ounce. The most crucial step in figuring pizza calories is **weighing** the slices. An average slice weighs four ounces. If you love to eat pizza, but don't want the calories, select a vegetarian pizza *without* the cheese. Don't knock it until you've tried it. Sprinkle several tablespoons of Parmesan cheese (30 calories per tablespoon) on top. At only 50 calories per ounce, three 4-oz. slices amount to 600 calories instead of 1000.

Weighing Food

The next time you are in the produce department of your favorite grocery store, choose an apple and place it on the scale. Compare a four-ounce apple to an eight-ounce one. Find a 10-ounce potato. At 20 calories per ounce that's 200 calories. Ten ounces of French fries supply 900. Weigh a bunch of grapes, cherries or green beans. How much does it take to make a pound? Experiment at home with cookies, crackers, cereals and breads. How many make one ounce? Soon you will be able to attach a number to every food.

Foods That Cannot Be Weighed

Obviously, some foods, like soups, casseroles, and pasta dishes, can not be weighed. In these cases, ask yourself, "Is it oily or buttery?" Take broccoli soup, for example, "Is it prepared with cream or milk?" If it's cream, then it is high in fat. A pasta dish that contains a cheese or oil-based sauce is higher fat than one prepared in a wine or tomato-based sauce. Determine the ingredients in the recipe, then use the calorie barometer to judge whether this is a good choice for you.

Beverages are, obviously, another food source that can not be weighed. These can be figured by **fluid** ounce.

They have their own barometer that looks like this:

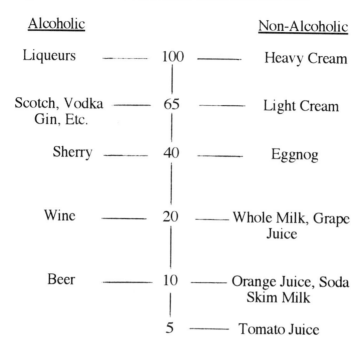

Alcoholic				Non-Alcoholic
Liqueurs	——	100	——	Heavy Cream
Scotch, Vodka Gin, Etc.	——	65	——	Light Cream
Sherry	——	40	——	Eggnog
Wine	——	20	——	Whole Milk, Grape Juice
Beer	——	10	——	Orange Juice, Soda Skim Milk
		5	——	Tomato Juice

From this point, multiply the number of ounces by the calories per ounce. For example, a six-ounce glass of white wine would supply 120 calories. Red wines and champagne are actually a bit higher at 25 calories per ounce. An eight ounce glass of whole milk yields 160 calories. And a one and a half ounce shot of vodka supplies approximately 100 calories. Measure the number of ounces your drinking glasses contain. Even something as innocent as fruit juice can add up in calories.

Tablespoons Matter

Certain condiments have been mentioned earlier in the chapter, but to give you a more complete rundown, note the barometer for tablespoons.

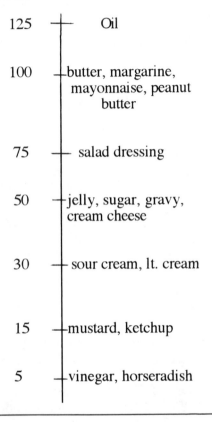

125	Oil
100	butter, margarine, mayonnaise, peanut butter
75	salad dressing
50	jelly, sugar, gravy, cream cheese
30	sour cream, lt. cream
15	mustard, ketchup
5	vinegar, horseradish

Spend the next couple of weeks learning the numbers on the barometers and applying them to the foods you eat. Record the food you eat and calculate the calories. You may be amazed at what you learn. In a short time you will become no less than a calorie expert.

THE CALORIE BAROMETER

Calories Per Ounce

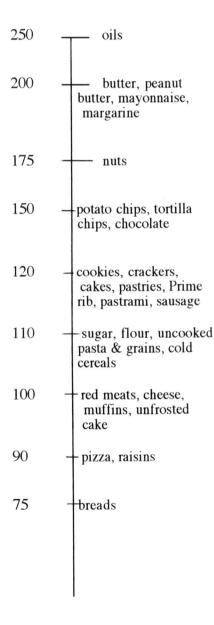

250 — oils

200 — butter, peanut butter, mayonnaise, margarine

175 — nuts

150 — potato chips, tortilla chips, chocolate

120 — cookies, crackers, cakes, pastries, Prime rib, pastrami, sausage

110 — sugar, flour, uncooked pasta & grains, cold cereals

100 — red meats, cheese, muffins, unfrosted cake

90 — pizza, raisins

75 — breads

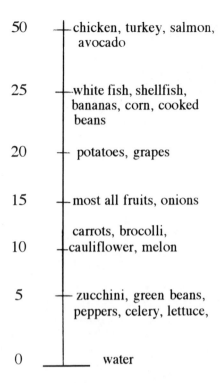

50 — chicken, turkey, salmon, avocado

25 — white fish, shellfish, bananas, corn, cooked beans

20 — potatoes, grapes

15 — most all fruits, onions

10 — carrots, brocolli, cauliflower, melon

5 — zucchini, green beans, peppers, celery, lettuce,

0 — water

6 Master Your Environment

Everyone dreams of a day when they can take a pill that allows them to eat unlimited pizza, burgers, and ice cream without the consequences. Unfortunately, the reality is, no drug will ever wipe out the effects of a diet high in saturated fats and a lifestyle lacking in physical activity. So, what are your options? It's got very little to do with willpower. The power is in learning to **master your environment**.

There are two simple steps to mastering your environment: The first step is taking an inventory of your current situation. The second step is creating accountability. To take an inventory, examine your kitchen: Inside your cupboards, pantry, freezer, and refrigerator. Which foods are the ones that you have no business buying in the first place, if you want to get fit and healthy? Be honest. Do your children really need double chocolate-chip cookies when they come home from school? Are nacho-flavored chips the healthiest snack you can think of?

Remember, what is most available, is what one eats. It's time to weed out the saturated fat and embrace the healthy, lowfat choices. Try keeping a colorful bowl of fresh fruit on your kitchen table. If it's in front of you, you have a greater chance of eating it. If fresh fruit is not available, then opt for frozen. (Just store it in the freezer.) Make smoothies with lowfat yogurt and a banana. Keep pre-cut, pre-washed salad ingredients in your frig for quick salads. Make a large bowl of popcorn when you feel like munching. Stock your shelves with pretzels, rice cakes, and no-fat crackers. Purchase some of those grains you've never tried before, like millet, couscous, barley, quinoa, or wheat bulgar. Eating a variety of grains will help you get all the different vitamins and minerals you need. Take your mother's spaghetti sauce recipe and "de-fat" it. Invest in a cookbook that offers simple ways of preparing Thai or Middle Eastern Food. Be adventurous.

When you food shop avoid the aisles that shelve cookies, chips and other prepackaged junk food, This way your inclination to buy them will be lessened. Don't buy junk for your children either. Teach them how to make healthy choices early on in their lives.

Buy oatmeal, barley, or a multi-grain hot cereal, instead of cold cereals. Go ahead, put brown sugar or honey on top. Nothing fills you up and makes you feel more satisfied on a cold morning than a generous bowl of hot cereal. When choosing bread, select a hearty <u>whole</u> grain loaf. Or make your own from scratch. Skip the butter and spread a fancy jam on top.

If you prefer to cook with oil, make it olive or canola oil and use it sparingly. For a naturally fat-free vegetable sauté use a combination of low-sodium tamari or soy sauce, apple juice and white wine. (This is my secret formula, and it tastes great.) Spices are fat-free and great flavor-enhancers, so use these freely. Purchase a collection of tangy, sweet mustards to spice up poultry, sandwiches or vegetables.

If you eat red meats, choose the leanest cuts of beef, lamb and pork. The term, "lean" *means less than 10 grams of fat per serving* and refers to red meat, poultry, and game meats. "Extra lean" means *less than five grams of fat per serving.* Stock up on skinless chicken breasts and lean ground turkey. Eat fish at least once a week.

Read labels on packaged foods. The first item listed in the ingredients is the one of which the food contains most. And each one thereafter contains progressively less. Avoid foods that contain coconut or palm oil which are the most saturated of fats.

Stay away from carbonated drinks, which create water retention. Drink plenty of fresh water, remember two quarts a day is recommended. Commercial juices are highly concentrated in sugar, so dilute them with water.

Be a list maker. You've heard the saying, "Don't go to the grocery store hungry." Don't go without a list either. Then, purchase *only* the items on the list.

Out in the *Real* World

You've stocked your fridge with fruits and vegetables. Your freezer contains two weeks-worth of your favorite lowfat entree. You've subscribed to a lowfat gourmet cooking magazine, and then, the weekend rolls around. Destination: Mexican Food.

Seated at your favorite South-of-the-border restaurant, your honorable intentions of eating healthy and lowfat are washed down with an icy Margarita. The basket of fresh tortilla chips lying casually on the table is now open game. You order the usual: chili rellenos served with refried beans, rice, extra guacamole and sour cream and, of course, another Margarita.

After the good time ends, you hate yourself and decide it's impossible to enjoy restaurant dining without compromising health and fitness.

This is what you did:

FOOD	FAT GRAMS	CALORIES*
1/2 basket of fried tortilla chips (2 oz.)	14	300
2 small margaritas	0	480
Chili Rellenos	22	425
1/2 cup beans (refried)	7	200
1/2 cup Mexican rice	6	125

2 T sour cream	5	60
2 T guacamole	6	80
TOTAL	60	1670

*These numbers are based on averages.

For a 150-pound woman, this meal consumes her total maintenance calories for the *entire* day. And exceeds a 20% fat diet by 26 grams.

Is it even possible to eat a lowfat, healthy meal at a Mexican restaurant? Or any restaurant, for that matter? Yes. Below is an alternative scenario that promotes health without deprivation. Could you live with this?

FOOD	FAT GRAMS	CALORIES
steamed corn tortillas (2 oz)	0	120
one light beer	0	100
1 chicken tostada* or fajita	8	200
served with 1/2 c. whole beans	0	125
and vegetables	0	50
1/2 cup Mexican rice	6	125
2 T sour cream	5	60
2 T salsa	0	30
TOTAL	19	710

*Do not eat the shell

Notice that the amount of food has not been reduced, but the calories have been cut in half and fat content decreased by two thirds.

Determine Your Destiny

As previously demonstrated, simply walking into a restaurant can be the beginning of the end for those attempting to eat healthy. To be successful, it is important to incorporate certain procedures. Scan the menu before you sit down and decide whether there is a high probability of overeating. Once seated, choosing lowfat foods depends a lot on communicating well with your food server and developing an assertive style of ordering. Don't be afraid to ask how a certain dish is prepared. If it contains oil or butter, ask to have it steamed, broiled, or baked. Suggest cooking in wine, spices, or soy sauce as an alternative to oil or butter. Always ask if lower fat foods may be substituted for high fat ones. For example, substitute a green salad or baked potato for French fries or potato salad. If this can not be done, then completely omit the high fat item.

If your broiled swordfish arrives drenched in butter, or your turkey sandwich slathered in mayonnaise, courteously ask that it be returned, and your request be honored. You may not win a popularity contest with the food server, but remember, this is about **your** health. If you feel like you're being too obnoxious, compensate by leaving a better tip. Another trick is ordering from the appetizer menu. A large bowl of soup (water or tomato-based) and a shrimp cocktail or specialty salad served with fresh French bread (without butter) provide an excellent lowfat, tasty, and satisfying meal. Always ask for sauces and dressings to be served on the side, so you can control the amounts.

The following examples and suggestions are designed to help you dine out successfully. Don't hesitate to add your own ideas.

MEXICAN

<u>PITFALLS</u>:
    *Basket of chips on the table.
    *Wide selection of fried foods: chimichangas,
        taquitos, chilis rellenos, refried beans.

<u>SOLUTIONS / OPTIONS</u>:
    *Ask for the chips to be removed and order a basket
        of fresh steamed corn tortillas.
    *Order dishes prepared without fat. Those served in
        red enchilada or green chili sauce are
        OK.
    *Substitute whole beans for the refried.
    Try these:
        -chicken or shrimp fajitas
        -tostada or burrito with whole beans or
        chicken, extra veggies and no cheese

ITALIAN

<u>PITFALLS</u>:
    *Bread served with olive oil; Antipastas that
        include cheese, high-fat meats, and
        vegetables marinated in oil.
    *A complicated menu.
    *High-fat sauces: Alfredo, pesto, meat,   and
        cheese sauces.
    *High-fat gelato, ice creams, and pastries.

<u>SOLUTIONS / OPTIONS</u>:
    *Ask for bread to be served **with** your meal
        and without butter or olive oil. Order a salad
        with dressing on the side, and use it
        sparingly.
    *Ask your server to recommend a lowfat
        dish or inquire about the ingredients of one
        with which you're unfamiliar.

*Choose pastas in tomato, marinara, wine, or
white clam sauces. Sprinkle with Parmesan
cheese.
*Order vegetarian pizza without cheese.
*Sprinkle with Parmesan cheese.
*For dessert order a refreshing fat-free sorbet.

CHINESE

PITFALLS:
*Most selections are sautéed in lots of oil.
*Appetizers such as egg rolls, pot stickers, and won
tons are all deep-fried.
*Most dishes are served family style, which may
lead to overeating.

SOLUTIONS / OPTIONS
*Order your selection prepared without oil.
*Suggest the use of soy sauce, broth, or water.
(The pans in which these foods are cooked
have been well seasoned. You will be
amazed how delicious the foods taste without
the oil.)
*Avoid selections that contain peanuts or cashews.
Forget sweet-and-sour pork, since the
pork is deep fried.
Try pot sticker steamed instead of fried.
Order steamed rice, not fried.

Accountability

You are now ready for the second part of mastering your
environment: Accountability. This is achieved by keeping
food records. By keeping account of the foods you eat for a
couple of weeks, you will learn more about calories, fat,
food choices, and how these impact your fitness and health,
than by engaging in *any* other health management activity.

This is not only a potent tool, but a commitment much easier than eating a rigid diet. And believe it or not, it only takes a few minutes a day. To begin you'll need the following equipment:

    1. A spiral note pad that fits easily into your purse or pocket. This you will carry with you wherever you go. Be sure it is not too big to tote or too small to write in comfortably. Otherwise you may well create a barrier to your success.

    2. A food scale that weighs up to one or two pounds.

    3. A completed Calorie Barometer (page 67)

Keeping a Food Journal

The most accurate records are kept by writing down every morsel of food you eat within 15 minutes. If you wait until the end of the day, chances are you will forget a greater portion of your intake. Weigh foods whenever possible, then, using the calorie barometer, record an estimated number of calories.

Resistance

At first, keeping a record of the food you eat may seem like a monumental task, and you may be thinking, "forget this!" In fact, I could probably write an entire book on the excuses people devise for not keeping records. The point of keeping a food journal is to help you make changes that will support health and fitness. However, I do understand the opposition. It isn't easy to confront our behavior, especially after eating things like cheeseburger, fries or chocolate covered donuts. In fact, this is usually when the commitments go down the tubes and the promises about "tomorrow" kick in. But are we really fooling ourselves by avoiding our behavior? Remember, every excuse you make is an excuse for being unfit and unhealthy. A food journal helps you create a food plan that supports your goals. Without record of your behavior, you continue to live in denial.

I once had a client, who after successfully losing 50 pounds, was walking three miles five days a week, and eating a lowfat diet with plenty of fruits, vegetables and grains. But for *some* reason, she was gaining weight. The only procedure she resisted was keeping a food journal.

As the weeks passed, the scale kept going up. Together, she and I reconstructed everything she had eaten (that she could remember) for one week. One item that kept coming up for breakfast was a cinnamon roll.

The following day I went to the bakery where she purchased these cinnamon rolls. Just by looking at them, I knew what the problem was. I brought one home and put it on the food scale. It registered **eight and a half ounces**! At 120 calories per ounce, this baby supplied over 1000 calories, nearly 60 grams of fat and two thirds of my client's daily maintenance calories. No wonder she was gaining weight. After this, it didn't take much convincing to get her to weigh, measure and <u>record</u> the foods she ate. And the cinnamon rolls dropped off her menu.

Awareness

By keeping records you become aware. Let's look at a sample of Jane's food records <u>before</u> she made any changes:

4 oz. croissant	500 calories
1/2 T butter	50
coffee, black	0
roast beef sandwich	600
w/ mayonnaise	100
1 small bag chips	225
soda	100

Fetticini Alfredo	550
2 oz. Fr. bread	150
1/2 T butter	50
Caesar salad	400
coffee, black	0
Grand Total	2725

Compare that to her new menu:

4 oz. bagel	320 calories
1 T. blackberry jam	50
1/4 (5 oz.) cantaloupe	50
coffee, black	0

turkey sandwich	400
w/ mustard	15
1/2 pint Cole slaw	125
1 bag (3 cups) popcorn	125
flavored mineral water	0

Linguini and red	
clam sauce	250
2 oz. Fr. bread	150
house salad	30
w/ 2T lowfat dressing	60
1 glass white wine	100
vanilla ice cream	175
Grand Total	1850

By increasing fruits and vegetables and decreasing fat, Jane reduced her calories by nearly 900. A change like this only three days a week, makes a difference of forty pounds of fat over one year.

Progress, Not Perfection

Use your food journal to set goals. For example, monitor the number of fruits and vegetables you eat per day by reviewing the previous two weeks of records and counting them. If you counted less than five, you've got work to do. If you counted five, try increasing it to seven. Remember, one piece of fruit or a half cup of vegetables furnishes one serving.

To achieve the recommended 60-65% carbohydrate diet, include four to six servings of bread, pasta, rice, cereal, or other grains per day. One piece of bread, 1/2 cup of rice, 3/4 cup pasta or cereal, or 1/2 a bagel provide one serving. Each serving supplies roughly 100 calories.

If your natural tendency is to judge yourself, try, instead, to have tolerance, even compassion, for yourself as you learn to eat healthier foods. No one learns anything by being perfect, so be prepared to make mistakes. Just don't make the mistake of NOT writing down the food you have eaten. Whether it's two celery sticks or three bear claws, write it down. After that, don't forget to put the number of calories next to it.

Continue with your record keeping behavior for as long as it takes to master your environment. Record keeping is one of your greatest teachers. And remember, your environment is more important than willpower. Reflect on what you have learned about your eating behaviors. Look back at a week's worth of eating and ask yourself: What did I learn about my food patterns? What success did I have? Congratulate yourself on your efforts and go forward. No matter what, don't give up. You are in the process of learning a new lifestyle.

7 Telling the Truth

In the last five chapters you have learned about specific behaviors, necessary facts and valuable skills that promote health and fitness. Yet, even the most effective strategies will lose their impact if you are eating for unresolved emotional issues.

What's Food Got to Do With It?

Between 80 and 100 million people in the United States have a weight problem. Of those who *do* manage to lose weight, 98% regain it all. Nearly thirty percent of all college-age women admit that they engaged in some form of bingeing, purging or starving themselves. With statistics like these, it seems that something much deeper than overeating and not exercising is going on.

As women, we face a double bind. Throughout history our job has been to shop, cook, and feed those we love. We're supposed to be polite, friendly, and selfless. We repress feelings that we believe cause us to appear "unfeminine" or "unattractive." Judged by our appearances, we have been fed a lie that our minds and our inner resources are not valuable. This false belief compels us to use our looks to gain power. And in doing so, we forsake ourselves, suffering deep emotional consequences, such as depression and self-hatred. Look at the number of women who now go under the knife for cosmetic surgery. American women spend more than $8 billion annually[1] on surgical procedures, many for no other reason than to conform to a specific standard of beauty. An increasing number of women are turning to anti-depressants[2], sleeping pills and anti-anxiety drugs, just to get through the day (and night.)

Most people eat for reasons other than hunger. Anger, boredom, disappointment, loneliness, and stress are just a few of those reasons. I believe that obesity, and in a large part, even cancer and heart disease, are all caused by a sickness that goes much deeper than eating high-fat foods and not exercising.

The diet and fitness industries, making over $30 billion a year, have offered a magnitude of sound **and** not-so-sound solutions. True, to achieve health and fitness success, we need to eat less fat and increase our physical activity, but do we need to consume pills, powdered formulas and prepackaged foods? Perhaps we have been brainwashed into thinking so. Are our metabolisms really defective? Have our bodies betrayed us? Do we, in fact, need a substance outside ourselves to be acceptable? No. No, to all of the above. No supplement, medical procedure, or diet can provide us with the acceptance, comfort, or happiness that we crave, but believe we don't deserve. The real issues have little, perhaps even *nothing*, to do with food. The real issues are connected with telling the truth about who we are and how we feel. Haven't we lied to ourselves long enough?

When you tell a lie, your heart races, your stomach tightens and the palms of your hands sweat. It's no secret that our bodies are intricately connected to our mind and emotions.[3] This is the premise upon which lie detector tests operate. What then happens to your body each time you suppress your truth by turning to food? Perhaps you have shoved your truth so far down inside that you don't even know it exists.

We need to see ourselves as more than just bodies. Every time we do not cherish ourselves as precious beings of love, truth and wisdom, we continue to buy into the lie that "if only I lost weight, my life would suddenly become perfect." When we believe our weight is the cause of our unhappiness, then we avoid looking at the *real* reasons for our problems. When we're thinking about what to eat next, we don't feel the fear. When we're planning how to lose the next 20 pounds, we don't feel the shame. And when we're totally immersed in how we look, there is no time to feel the anger or sadness.

Patterns From The Past

If the practice of using food as a coping method no longer serves you, then it may be time to explore the patterns from your past. This is not an attempt to blame anyone, but an opportunity to see from where certain beliefs originate.

Imagine yourself as a tiny baby: When hungry, you cried; Someone, usually your mother, came to feed you. While fed, you were held and cuddled. Your basic needs were met. As a toddler, you learned to sit in your high chair. As you grew into a preschooler, you learned about manners. You were praised for using your fork and scolded for using your fingers. You were introduced to the world of socialization. Perhaps your family members shared their laughter and joy as the meat and potatoes were passed around the dinner table. Or maybe, anger and tension brewed as the butter was spread upon the bread. In which case, meals may have been a time of confusion or even fear. It may have been at this time that food became the glue that kept your emotions intact.

The following exercise may help you discover your feelings and beliefs associated with food:

Find a safe, quiet, and private location where you can let go of pending responsibilities. You may choose a den, a sunny bedroom, or a place outside amongst the trees and under the sky. Wherever it is, be sure to free yourself of any restrictions or rules that you may ordinarily place upon yourself. When you feel comfortable with your special location, provide yourself with paper and a writing tool. Choose colorful paper or poster board; Crayons or markers. When you are ready to begin, close your eyes and let your imagination flow. You are about to take a journey back in time.

Imagine yourself as a child of five or six. You are skipping happily along a beautiful tree-lined road on a warm afternoon. Birds are singing and there is a gentle breeze. As you wander down the road, you see a familiar scene in the distance: The home you grew up in. You are drawn towards it. The sun is beginning to set and the lights inside the house are aglow. You smell the aroma of your mother's (father's or grandma's) cooking and walk up to the front door. You hesitate at first, but then step inside. As you advance towards the kitchen you hear the conversation and you remember all the meals you shared with your family. As you glance towards the kitchen table, you notice everyone in your family is seated there. They invite you to join them. You decide to sit down in the special chair that was always saved just for you. You may recognize the design of the wallpaper, the clock on the wall above the sink, the checkered curtains or the face on the cookie jar. And as these memories fill your mind's eye, what feelings fill your soul? Are you happy and relaxed? Or are you distressed and tense? Do you speak? If so, are you heard? What are the dynamics between you and the others? How do you feel about the food being served? Does your mouth water as you wait for a slice of roasted chicken or do you turn your nose up at the stuffed peppers? Do you calmly chew your food or do you shovel it in and swallow it half chewed? Observe every detail. And feel all the emotions that you may have repressed back then. If a smile crosses your lips, don't hold it back. If tears well up in your eyes, let them tumble down your cheeks. If this feels like too much to deal with, remember you can always come back to the present with a blink of your eyes. When you sense you have spent enough time here, you can step away from the table and say your good-byes. As you leave, take one last look at the room filled with its memories. How does it feel to walk away? Are you sad? Anxious? Happy? Relieved? When you are ready to return to the present take a deep breath and gradually open your eyes.

Now, with your drawing materials, create a picture that describes your experience. Draw. Scribble. Print. Do whatever comes to mind. Let your picture tell a story. If a picture doesn't come to you, then write down your experience in words. When you have completed this, take a moment to create some distance from your experience. And then come back to it at a later time to observe how this experience is linked to your present relationship with food.

During this exercise in my workshops, several women found themselves at their grandmother's houses, where they felt safer than at their own homes. Others noticed how they felt compelled to clear the table before they left. Still others flatly refused to go inside.

One woman, I'll call Anne, remembered her mother's beef stew, which she utterly abhorred. One of the rules of the house was to eat everything on your plate, even if you weren't hungry. Her mother would always say, "There are starving children in Africa." As an adult, Anne finished every bite of food on her plate, whether she was hungry or not. Becoming aware of this connection helped her realize that now, as an adult, she had the power to change her behavior.

Jennifer, another woman, drew a picture of a watermelon surrounded by many happy faces. Her own face, she drew in a black cloud, separate from the others. During her childhood in Missouri, on the hot summer nights, her father would bring home a huge, freshly picked watermelon. Her mother would line the kitchen table with newspapers and cut the melon down the middle, slicing off triangular pieces. Then, Jennifer and her family would sit around the table enjoying the melon and each other's company as they spit the seeds out onto the paper-lined table. She believed her security would never be threatened. But then, when Jennifer, who was the youngest child, turned ten years old, her mother died suddenly of a heart attack. After this, her father emotionally withdrew from the family and her siblings drifted apart. Jennifer was never able to grieve her mother's death. To deal with her sorrow she ate. Food became the friend that would never leave or disappoint her. Realizing this, Jennifer decided it was time to do the grieving she had never done. By seeking the counsel of a therapist she was able to release her long repressed sadness. And by doing this healing work, she no longer needed to medicate her feelings with food.

Debbie, who came from an alcoholic home, drew a crowd of angry faces around her dining room table with her own face positioned in the middle. Words like "Chew with your mouth shut!" "Use your napkin!" "Don't spill your milk!" were coming from their mouths. A sample of her illustration is pictured next:

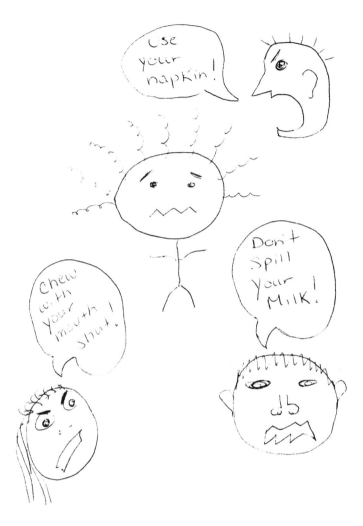

Her family members had always expressed criticisms of one another at the dinner table and Debbie's weight was a popular topic. As a result, she felt angry, self-conscious and began to secretly binge. What she realized by doing this exercise was that her weight seemed to be directly proportional to the amount of anger she stuffed. With the help of a professional, she learned she had a right to express her anger and that her weight was no one's business but her own. The more she identified and appropriately expressed her anger, the less she binged.

What issues came up for you during the visualization? How can you change your belief system to more accurately match your present reality? Share this with a trustworthy friend or counselor. And remember, healing takes time, don't expect yourself to change overnight.

When Feelings Were Expressed

There was a time when we knew how to express our feelings freely. We cried when we were sad. We stomped our feet and said "No!" when we were angry. We may have sung or danced in delight when we were joyous. And then, sometime later in our lives we learned to shut down. We were convinced that crying was for babies and expressing anger was for bullies. We were rewarded for acting "good" and shamed for saying, "No." We choked down our tears, cut off our rage, and stopped telling the truth.

"The only way out is through."
Fritz Perlz

Picture a woman who drinks alcohol to prevent her pain from surfacing. She knows that her drinking is a problem, and from time to time she vows to never drink again. At first she succeeds, but when her feelings become intolerable, she returns to alcohol to anesthetize the pain. Consequently, her feelings submerge even deeper. The problem is, these feelings don't go away. Unexpressed feelings are like monsters in the closet. The more we try to pretend they aren't there, the bigger and more frightening they become. To make the monsters disappear, we hide under the covers. Alcohol represents the covers for the alcoholic. Food represents the covers for the obsessive dieter or compulsive overeater.

To come out from under the covers, you need to believe that you can walk through your pain, and not only *survive*, but **triumph**. You do this by discovering, expressing, and ultimately healing the long-buried feelings of abandonment, anger, loss, or neglect. Unfortunately, there are no guidelines or recommendations for the prevention of compulsive overeating as there are for cancer, heart disease and diabetes. There are no graphs that can measure the quantity of pain you "stuff" when you use food as an anesthetic. Learning to express your feelings (even though you may have grown up believing this was inappropriate) is the beginning of the journey toward healing.

It may be difficult to grieve, when you were told there was "no reason to cry." Or very uncomfortable to express anger, when you thought women were supposed to act "nice." Your task, if you choose to accept it, is to begin to acknowledge the fear, the panic, the despair. Give voice to the pain, the rage, the grief. Express that which has been locked up inside, one step at a time. This is what it means to tell the truth.

Declare Your Feelings

Have you ever noticed how exhausting it is, both physically and emotionally, to repress your feelings? Try to imagine, without judgment, what would happen if you let go and expressed your feelings?

ANGER: Anger is energy that must be released or it will implode, causing innumerable physical and emotional consequences. Most people have a hard time dealing with their anger and would prefer that it just "go away." However, unexpressed anger usually turns into migraines, ulcers, depression and, perhaps, even those so-called mystery diseases, such as chronic fatigue syndrome and fibromyalgia. During my work with patients restricted to a 500-calorie-a-day medically-supervised program, I noticed that many of them had become angry. Were they angry because they were not eating? Or had they, in the past, been repressing this anger **by** eating? Perhaps, by not eating, their anger finally had an opportunity to rear its head.

If you feel as though you are bottled-up with anger, I urge you to try releasing it. I once learned a technique for releasing anger from a wise psychotherapist. It is called "beating a pillow." I remember the first time she recommended this, I thought, "how crazy does she think I am?" But after putting aside my judgment, I found out that this method really works.

Choose a large pillow and a private location. (A closet has worked for me.) Hit the pillow in whatever fashion suits you and as you do, verbalize your anger. You might say, "I'm angry!" or "How dare you!" At the start, you may be unclear about why you are angry, because you have become such a master at concealing it. But after a few seconds of your fists hitting the pillow, you may be amazed to discover what comes up. Usually underneath the simmering rage awaits sadness or disappointment. Or you may blurt out unrehearsed words that have been locked up inside your subconscious for many years. By staying with your feelings, you may discover that you will not only survive, but you will also give birth to a part of yourself you forgot existed. A very strong part.

Beating a pillow is not the only method of releasing anger. I've heard of people hitting a punching bag, or doing some form of vigorous exercise, even housework. One word of caution: Physical or verbal abuse toward another person is **not** OK. In fact, this is usually a sign that you have an overload of unreleased feelings from the past.

SADNESS: Do any of these sayings sound familiar?

> "Don't cry over spilled milk."
> "Big boys/girls don't cry."
> "Crying doesn't change anything."
> "If you don't stop crying, I'll give you something to cry about!"

What is so burdensome to us, as a society, about expressing sorrow? Our culture's intolerance of tears became more evident to me once I had children. I remember thinking that my children shouldn't cry in public because it was an indication that something was wrong with me or my parenting skills. But when a woman in a department store turned to me in frustration because my two year-old was crying and said "can't you shut your kid up," I **woke** up. Children cry to express anger, sadness, frustration or disappointment. The more you try to stop a child from crying, the more the tears flow. Tears produce a chemically cleansing and healing effect on the body. Shedding tears is one of the ways our bodies are telling the truth.

I wonder how much healthier we, adults, would be if we gave ourselves the luxury of shedding our tears whenever we felt the need. How much less dependence on drugs, alcohol and food would there be if we learned to acknowledge and express our pain?

When my brother died of cancer several years ago, I grieved for many months. The more I let myself cry and express my grief (with **safe**, **caring** people) the better I was able to deal with my loss. The next time you watch a sad movie or find yourself in a situation that causes your throat to tighten and your eyes to sting, let it out. Sob. Tremble. Let your tears wash away the pain. After the storm has passed, you may discover an incredibly healing calm. (If you are seriously depressed or suicidal, you need to seek professional help. Find listings for grief counseling and suicide-prevention programs in your telephone directory.)

FEAR: When you were a child, you may have been afraid of the dark. Perhaps a night-light helped dispel your fears. Or you may have needed your mom or dad to hold you and tell you that everything was safe. But if someone told you that your fears were ridiculous, then you probably learned to discount those feelings early on. Most women who have an overwhelming fear of being "fat" use this to mask deeper fears. By learning to acknowledge and embrace our fears, we can begin to dispel them. One way to do this is by keeping a "fear" journal. Everyday, keep account of your fears as they surface. Your journal might look something like this:

> *I'm afraid I'm not enough.
> *I'm afraid I'll make a mistake.
> *I'm afraid I'll let someone down.
> *I'm afraid of intimacy.
> *I'm afraid of looking stupid.
> *I'm afraid I won't be accepted.

After you've written down your fears, ask yourself where they come from. Who told you that you weren't enough? What experiences caused you to fear intimacy? This is another opportunity to look into the patterns of your past to find some answers. Working with a professional on this is recommended. Ultimately, when we live in fear, we are not fully living.

Getting Support

In a society of dysfunction and fear, where families are broken or dispersed throughout the country, we need to connect with others. By getting support, we experience a powerful element of healing. Many people believe that they have to solve their problems on their own. but we all need and deserve support.

Studies indicate that recovering cancer patients sharply increase their survival rate when they join and participate in group support. Without support, problems can loom larger as hopelessness and isolation proliferate. Without a network of support we often turn to inappropriate ways of coping with our problems. When choosing the type of support that best satisfies your needs, consider both group and individual options.

Group support, offers a safe environment where one can relate her feelings and issues to other people who understand. Currently popular are the Twelve-Step groups which have over 60 years of a successful track record.

These groups, founded as Alcoholics Anonymous, now address other problems, such as overeating, gambling and relationship addictions. Each of these groups provide a unique, nonjudgmental setting where one's problems and feelings can be expressed "anonymously." When we can shed our shame, it becomes safe to share our feelings and reveal our authentic selves. And once we do this, our addictions lessen and eventually end.

If Twelve-Step Programs don't sound right for you, try a women's support group, a church-affiliated group or call your local hospital for a list of groups available in your area. For some people individual counseling may be a more comfortable option than group support. If this is the case for you, choose a professional with whom you feel safe: A trained, licensed marriage and family counselor, a licensed social worker, or, perhaps, the pastor of your church.

Case Study

Alexis had been a prisoner of her eating disorder for nearly ten years before she came into a support group. Ever since she was a preschooler, her mother had told her that "a girl should be pretty, have a good figure, and act sweet" - only in this way would she attract a man." (Which according to Alexis's mother, was the only reason to exist.) Her mother had been raised by very abusive parents, so getting married had been her saving grace.

At the age of nine, Alexis showed a deep interest and talent in art. Her schoolteachers encouraged her to draw and paint, but her mother told her that art was a waste of time. As the years progressed, Alexis found her only solace in food, and as a result, she gained a lot of weight. To alleviate the shame she felt being fat, and her mother's unbearable pressure, she devised what she believed to be a secret method for losing the weight: self-induced vomiting.

By her nineteenth birthday, Alexis had learned her mother's lesson well: She had already received three marriage proposals. Finally at the age of twenty-two she accepted one. For seven years she had practiced her eating disorder. Even after her wedding the bingeing and purging remained a constant daily ritual. It took less than six months before her new husband's alcoholism became evident. As did his physical and emotional abuse. A broken marriage was a family taboo, so Alexis tolerated her husband's abuse for three years. It wasn't until she went to the emergency room with a broken jaw that she was convinced she needed to take action. The emergency room staff directed her to a safe shelter for battered women and there, she attended a support group.

At her first meeting she felt a sense of relief. She was awed by the openness and honesty of the women. She didn't say a word for the first three weeks. Then when she felt safe enough, she began to share her own feelings of fear, pain and worthlessness. The other members seemed to understand her pain. They acknowledged her feelings and offered her the kind of support she had never known. She discovered that she was not responsible for her husband's drinking and she didn't deserve his abuse. The more Alexis expressed her feelings, the less she felt compelled to binge and purge.

Before long she returned to painting and applied for a job at an art gallery. Along with divorce papers, she filed a restraining order against her husband and moved into her own apartment. A year later she was still attending her support group and was no longer bingeing and purging. She had finally learned to value who she was.

"There is no birth of consciousness without pain."
Carl Jung

You may shrink at the idea of expressing your "real" feelings because this means exposing your authentic self. And doing that can be terrifying. Why? Because to expose your authentic self means risking abandonment, disapproval, and rejection. Facing painful, uncomfortable feelings may cause overwhelming anxiety, even <u>more</u> anxiety than being unfit and unhealthy. To get in touch with your feelings, you need to reconnect with the precious being inside you.

The Precious Being Inside You

Have you forgotten how lovable, creative and full of life you were as a child? If so, it's time to remember. Locate a picture of yourself as a baby or toddler. Take a few moments to look into this child's eyes. Notice the details of this little person; The expression on her face; The position of her hands. What does the picture say about this child? What was going on for her at this time? What were her dreams? Her aspirations? Did she achieve them? What did happen?

Now bring your attention back to the present. Knowing that this precious being grew up and turned to food as a method of coping with her feelings, how would you comfort and nurture her? Obviously, you wouldn't criticize her for not being a size eight. Nor would you starve her until the scale registered a certain number. Would you give her a bag of chips and say, "Drown your sorrows in this?" I'm sure you wouldn't say or do any of these things to this child, right? So, then, why do you say and do these things to her now?

Take a minute, *this* minute, to write down five loving, supportive statements that you would like to tell her. For example,
"You are perfect just the way you are."
"You deserve happiness."
"You are loved."
"It is safe to feel your feelings."
"I will always be there for you."

If you find this difficult, I recommend reading one of the books on positive affirmations. Any title by Louise Hay is great. Another good one is *Positive Self-Talk for Children*, by Douglas Bloch.

Once you have completed your list, take each statement and change the "you" to an "I" statement.   So, the above examples would be:

"I am perfect just the way I am."

"I deserve happiness."

"I am loved" or, better yet, "I love myself."

"It is safe to feel my feelings."

"I will always be there for myself."

Then, each morning, choose one or two of these affirmations to say to yourself in the mirror. This may feel awkward at first because many women are so accustomed to berating themselves. Do it anyway. The emotionally starved little child that lives within you needs to hear these positive messages.

After you have completed the affirmations, make a list of the things this precious child would like to do. Perhaps she would like to take a hike in the mountains, have a picnic at the park, or play in the sand at the beach. Or maybe the teenager in you would love to get her nails manicured, take a bubble bath by candlelight, or eat breakfast in bed. Make a list of at least six things she would love to do. Then set a date, a time, and follow through with the plan.

By doing these things for this precious child, you are learning to love and nurture yourself. Many of us have been raised to believe we must take care of others and that taking care of ourselves is selfish, even sinful. But the truth is, without loving and taking care of ourselves first, we can not love or take care of anyone else. How do you show someone you love them? By spending time with them, feeding them healthy foods, allowing them to express themselves and praising them for their specialness. How would it feel to start treating yourself as someone you loved?

Finding the Inner Voice

Most of us are so busy with life's activities that we are totally disconnected from the inner voice of guidance that lives inside each of us. Meditation is an excellent opportunity to awaken our inner voice. In *The Tibetan Book of Living and Dying*, Sogyal Rinpoche writes, "Generally we waste our lives, distracted from our true selves, in endless activity; meditation, on the other hand, is the way to bring us back to ourselves, where we can really experience and taste our full being, beyond all habitual patterns[4]."

Meditation means taking the time to quiet our minds, relax our bodies and create inner peace. By shutting out the constant chatter in which our minds are trained to engage, the unconscious has an opportunity to reveal itself. In this way we have a chance to listen to the inner voice which is our inner truth. Meditation doesn't mean you have to lock yourself up in a closet and chant "om" for an hour. Nevertheless, if this is your choice, then go for it.

I remember the first time I tried to meditate; I decided to spend five minutes on what at the time seemed much like fruitless behavior. (But I'm always willing to try something once if it can help me.) I turned my kitchen timer on and rested comfortably on my couch with my eyes closed. Within seconds I was making a mental list of all the things I had to do that day. Then suddenly I noticed the sound of the timer clicking. "Why is that silly thing on?" I thought to myself. Then I remembered, I was trying to quiet my mind.

Since that first time, I now take thirty minutes from the hustle and stress of the day to meditate. It is during this quiet time that I often find an answer to a long-held question or a solution to a nagging problem. Other times, I just let go of pressing worries and concerns. Afterward, I feel refreshed and serene.

There are many wonderful books now available that can help you learn more about meditation and how to achieve the rewarding results. Check with your local bookstore or library.

Our Bodies Speak to U s

Much of what you have read about in this chapter will help you do what you may have avoided for many years ...

that is, listen to your body. Our bodies are giving us messages every moment, but we have learned to ignore them. For example, what do you do as soon as you feel a bit tired or lethargic? Most people reach for caffeine. How different might we feel if instead we took 10 minutes to close our eyes, breathe deeply and rest, drank a refreshing glass of juice, or took a ten minute walk. What other messages does your body give you? When you feel chilled, this is a message to put on a sweater. When you feel lonely, perhaps it's time to call or visit a friend. When you feel stressed and overwhelmed, maybe you need to spend time alone. Start listening to your body.

Pay attention to and express your feelings appropriately. Don't do it alone: you deserve to have support. Meditate everyday, even if it's only for five minutes. Trust your instincts, honor your courage and praise your efforts. Love yourself. Remember, all the answers lie within.

The following chapter is a collection of quick and simple, lowfat (and no-fat) recipes. Enjoy.

8 Twenty E-Z Lowfat Recipes

NANCY'S OATBRAN PANCAKES

2 oz. oatbran (1/2 cup dry)　　dash salt
1/2 cup buttermilk　　　　　　1 tsp. b. soda
2 egg whites
2 tsp. sugar

Let oatbran soak for 20-30 minutes in milk.
Stir in all other ingredients well.
Spray pan with cooking spray. Cook as you
would ordinary pancakes.
Serve with fruit or syrup.

NO-FAT CARROT BRAN MUFFINS

1 cup skim or 1 percent milk　　2 T. brown sugar
1 cup raisin bran cereal　　　　1 egg
1 cup whole wheat flour　　　　3 T. orange juice
$^1/_2$ cup oat bran　　　　　　　1 cup grated carrots
1 tsp. baking powder　　　　　1/2 cup dried fruit
$^1/_2$ tsp. baking soda
$^1/_4$ tsp. salt
$^1/_2$ tsp. cinnamon

Combine cereal and milk. Let stand for 5 minutes.
Combine dry ingredients. Put wet ingredients, except for the
carrots & fruits, in with the cereal. Add dry ingredients.
Mix well. Stir in carrots and raisins. Bake at 400° for 15 -
20 minutes in muffin tins sprayed with non-stick spray.

ZUCCHINI SOUP

1 strip bacon,
  (cooked, drained & crumbled)
1 T. olive oil   5 zucchini (chopped)
1 medium onion   1 can chicken broth
1 & 1/2 stalk celery   2 cups water
8 mushrooms   1/4 tsp. pepper
1 potato (peeled & chopped) 1 tsp. basil

Chop and sauté onion, celery and mushroom in olive oil.
Place potato & zucchini in saucepan with chicken broth,
water, pepper and basil. Add sautéed vegetables. Bring to
boil. Simmer 35 minutes. Take half of soup and puree,
then re-add to original mixture. Add bacon last for flavor.
(For vegetarians, omit bacon, add 1/2 tsp. salt.)

COUSCOUS SALAD

                                             Dressing:
1 1/4 cup broth or water   1/8 c. olive oil
1 cup couscous, dry   1/2 c. lemon juice
1/4 cup green onions   2 minced garlic
1/2 cup tomatoes   1 tsp. Dijon Mustard
1/4 cup parsley   1 tsp. gr. coriander
1/2 cup cucumbers   Salt & Pepper
1/4 cup grated carrots
1 /4 cup Feta cheese, crumbled

Bring water/broth to boil. Stir in couscous. Cover and
remove from heat. Let stand for 15 minutes. Chill.
Add vegetables. Mix dressing ingredients and add to
couscous/vegetable mixture. Top with Feta cheese.

GARDEN SALAD

4 -5 cups organic Romaine and Butter Lettuce,
1/4 cup cilantro
1/2 cup chopped celery
1/2 cup grated carrots
1 beet (* see below)
1/4 cup minced red onion
2 sliced (organic, if available) tomatoes

Tear lettuce. Add cilantro and celery. Toss carrots, beets onions and tomatoes on top for color.

* For best results: Previous to making salad, wrap beet in tin foil and bake 350° degrees till tender. Cool and peel, then cut up into small pieces.

Honey Mustard Dressing

1 T. honey	4 T. rice vinegar
2 T. Poupon mustard	Salt & Pepper
2 T. olive oil	1 T. Sesame Seeds

Mix honey, mustard & vinegar.
Add rest of ingredients
and mix thoroughly. Toss over salad.

LORETTE'S LOWFAT LASAGNA

1 pint lowfat ricotta cheese / 1 pint lowfat cottage cheese
2 eggs / 2 boxes frozen chopped spinach (thawed)
1 cup white wine or beef bouillon
1 cup chopped mushrooms
1 cup chopped onions
1/2 cup chopped green peppers
1 cup chopped broccoli or zucchini
12 ounces lasagna noodles
1 cup lowfat spaghetti sauce (your favorite brand)
1/2 cup parmesan cheese

Blend ricotta, cottage cheese and eggs together. Steam all vegetables (except spinach) in white wine or bouillon. Drain spinach and add to other veggies. Cook till tender. Cook noodles. Drain. Spray pan with non-stick spray. Layer noodles, veggies, noodles, cheese/egg mixture, then spaghetti sauce. Repeat layers. Sprinkle parmesan cheese on top. Bake at 350° for 20-30 min.

SAUTÉED TERIYAKI VEGETABLES

1/2 cup chopped red onion   1 cup broccoli
1/2 cup red pepper   2 cups chopped Swiss chard
1 cup sliced zucchini   1 cup sliced mushrooms
1 cup chopped cabbage   1/4 cup of teriyaki sauce
1 cup cut carrots   1/3 cup white wine
                                 1/3 cup apple juice

Heat wine, teriyaki sauce and apple juice on med-high in wok or pan. Add onions and peppers first and cook till almost tender. Add in the following order: Broccoli, zucchini, cabbage, carrots. Let these cook a while then add Swiss chard and mushrooms last. As liquid evaporates add water. Keep stirring as you cook. Serve over brown rice with grated Parmesan cheese on top.

RED LENTILS STEW

6 cups water
2 1/2 cup red lentils
2 T. Miso or one chicken bouillon
1/2 cup chopped yellow onion
2 medium red potatoes   3 cloves garlic
1/2 cup celery   pinch celery salt

Mix miso in cup of hot water until dissolved. Then add to large stew pot of water, along with lentils and the rest of the ingredients. This is a real easy recipe into which you can literally throw any kind of vegetable or spice that you choose. Cook 30 -35 min. over a low heat after initial boil. Serve with a whole wheat bread and a salad.

TASTY LOWFAT CHILI

1/2 cup chix broth
1/2 cup each chopped: onions, garlic, green peppers, red
      peppers, carrots, zucchini
1 can tomato sauce
2 cans kidney beans
2 can stewed tomatoes, Mexican style
1 lb. ground turkey
1/2 tsp. cumin, paprika and salt and pepper

Steam sauté veggies in pan. Remove from pan. Brown turkey. Transfer to large pot. Add veggies and the rest of the ingredients. Simmer 1-2 hours. Serve over brown rice with a dollop of sour cream. A spinach salad and corn bread is a healthy and delicious complement.

TAMARI CHICKEN & CHINESE NOODLES

1 pkg. Chinese noodles (found in produce dept.)
4 chicken breasts, (skinless, boneless)
1 1/2 cup broccoli, cut up
1/2 cup onions, cup up
2 -3 cloves garlic   1/4 tsp. ground ginger
1/4 c. sesame seeds   1/2 cup tamari sauce

Cut chicken in bite size chunks. Sauté in tamari sauce. Add water as tamari evaporates. Once chicken is cooked, remove from pan and set aside. Sauté onions, garlic, broccoli and ginger in remaining tamari sauce. Once tender, add cooked chicken.
Cook Chinese noodles according to directions. Drain noodles. Serve chicken and vegetables tossed over noodles. Sprinkle with sesame seeds.

NANCY'S LOWFAT SPAGHETTI SAUCE

1 large onion chopped   2 - 14 oz. can tomatoes
3 cloves garlic, chopped   1 - 8 oz can Hunts tomato
2 T olive oil   sauce
1 1/4 ground turkey
2T oregano

Sauté the first four ingredients until brown, then add tomatoes and tomato sauce. Cover and simmer three hours. You may add beef bouillon or leeks for added flavor.

DELICIOUS LOWFAT MEATLOAF

16 ounces ground turkey
1-1/2 cups chopped Swiss chard or 1 pkg. frozen spinach,
    (defrosted and drained)
1 cup Quaker Oats
1/2 cup chopped onion
2 eggs
1/2 cup lowfat cottage cheese
1/4 cup ketchup   1/4 cup low salt soy sauce
Several shakes of parsley and garlic salt

Mix turkey and chard (or spinach) well. Add all ingredients
except oats. Mix well. Add oats last and mix well.
Place in loaf pan. Bake at 375^0 degrees for 45 minutes to
one hour. (You may also place in muffin tins for individual
mini loafs. Freeze after cool. Take from freezer as needed.)

QUINOA CASSEROLE

Quinoa (pronounced "keen wa"), a grain which supplies all
eight essential amino acids, originated in the Peruvian
Andes. It has a nutty flavor and can be found in most health
food stores.

1 cup cooked quinoa   1/2 cup lowfat milk
1 cup cooked brown rice   2 tsp. parsley
3/4 chicken, cooked, cubed 1/2 cup, grated Jack
2 eggs   cheese

Beat eggs & milk in mixing bowl. Add the rest of
ingredients. Mix well. Cook in the microwave covered for
7 min. on high or bake 350° for 30 minutes till eggs cook
thoroughly.

SPINACH PIE

One 10 oz pkg. frozen chopped spinach
1/2 cup chopped onion
1/2 T olive oil
2/3 minced garlic cloves
3 eggs
1/4 cup nonfat milk
1/2 cup shredded mozzarella cheese
1/2 cup parmesan cheese
1/2 tsp. basil, 1/2 tsp. parsley
non-stick spray
1/4 cup wheat germ (optional)

Thaw and drain spinach. Sauté onion and garlic in oil till tender. Set aside. Combine eggs and milk. Mix well. Stir in spinach, cheeses, spices. Add onions and garlic. Spray quiche baking dish with non-stick spray. Sprinkle the wheat germ to cover sides and bottom. Pour mixture in pan. Bake at 350° for 25-30 minutes.

TRIPLE POTATOES

1 yam
1 sweet potato
2 -3 red potatoes
1/2 cup diced purple onion

Sauce:
1/2 cup low
   sodium soy sauce
1/2 cup white wine
3 T Poupon mustard

Slice potatoes and stand them up on their sides in shallow baking dish. Place onions on top and pure sauce over entire ingredients. Bake at 350° for 40 min. until tender.

ZUCCHINI FRITTATA

2 zucchini, sliced diagonally
2 cloves garlic
1 cup gr. onions, sliced
1 tsp. celery salt
1 tsp. celery salt
1/2 cup fresh parsley

2 cups Swiss chard
1/2 cup Parmesan
    cheese
1/2 cup Mozz. cheese
2 T olive oil
Salt & Pepper

Sauté all veggies in olive oil. Cook 5-7 min. Set Aside. In a separate bowl beat eggs, spices, and cheeses, Add to veggies. Put into baking dish. Bake at 350° for 30 min.

NUALA'S PEACH AND BLUEBERRY CRUMBLE

Topping:
3/4 cup wh. wheat flour
3/4 cup oats
1 tsp. baking powder
1/4 tsp. salt
1 tsp. cinnamon
1/2 cup brown sugar
1 egg
1 T. butter

Fruit:
 6 cups peaches
4 cups blueberries

Fresh or frozen fruit may be used. If using frozen, defrost and drain well. Other fruit combinations, such as peach/blackberry or apple/blueberry, may be used. Use your imagination. Mix topping ingredients in a food processor by hand, long enough to get a fine mealy texture. Layer peaches in a shallow baking dish. Add blueberries on top. Then top with the crumble topping. Bake at 375 ° for 45 - 55 minutes until topping is brown.
Note: If using other fruit, be sure to put the firmer fruit (such as apples, pears) on the bottom and softer fruit (such as berries, cherries) on top.

NO FAT HONEY/OATMEAL COOKIES

1 cup applesauce
1/2 cup sugar
1/2 cup honey
1 egg
1 tsp. vanilla

2 cups flour
1 tsp. baking soda
a pinch salt
1 1/2 cups whole oats
1/2 cup raisins

Optional: 1/2 cup raisin bran

Combine the first four ingredients, mix well. Combine next three ingredients separately. Sift together well. Add the dry ingredients, except for oats, to wet ingredients and stir till completely mixed. Stir in oats and 1/2 cup raisins. If dough is too moist stir in raisin bran cereal until it is the consistency for cookies. Bake at 350° for 10-12 minutes.

CRAZY CAKE

3 cup flour
1/4 c applesauce
2 c. sugar
2 tsp. vanilla
4 T. cocoa
2 tsp. soda

1 tsp. salt
1/4c vinegar
2 c. cold water

Sift dry ingredients together into a 9 x 13 in pan. Make 3 holes. Put the applesauce in one whole. Vinegar in another. Vanilla in the last one. Pour water over all. Stir well but do not beat. Bake at 350° for 40-45 min. Put a thin glaze of almond flavoring, powdered sugar and milk on top.

108

CHOCOLATE BROWNIE PIZZA DESSERT

1 No Fat Brownie Mix
1 8 oz pkg. Lowfat cream cheese
3 T orange juice
orange and kiwi slices

Prepare the brownie mix as directed except put mix on a pizza stone or in a shallow round pan. Bake and completely cool. Add orange juice to cream cheese and mix thoroughly. Spread over brownie and top with orange and kiwi slices. Cut into pizza wedges and serve.

Endnotes

Chapter Two--Numbers That Count

1 - National Research Council on Life Sciences, Food and Nutrition Board and Committee on Diet, *Health, Diet and Health, Implications for Reducing Chronic Disease Risk* US Government Printing Office, 1989, pg. 142-143

Chapter Three--Exercise: What, When, Where and How Much

1 - Brewster, L., and Jacobson, M., *The Changing American Diet*, Center for Science in the Public Interest, 1983
2 - Although excess LDL's and VLDL's are culprits of artery blockage, a certain amount are necessary for production of certain hormones and to strengthen cellular make-up.
3 - To find 60% of your maximal heart rate, subtract your age from 220, then multiply that number by .60
4 - American Diabetes Association, *A Word About Obesity*, 1987
5 - One calorie burned for every five stairs climbed.

Chapter Five--Food Calories: The Good, Bad and the Ugly

1 - All calorie values taken from US Government Handbook # 456
2 - Because of its high oil content, carrot cake contains 140 calories an ounce, even though carrots only contain 12 per ounce.
3 - Taken from the following:

a)Kaufman, William, *Calorie Counter for 6 Quick Loss Diets*, Jove Books, NY

b)*Calorie Counter & Menu Guide*, Dell Publishing, NY

c)The American Heart Association's *Fat and Cholesterol Counter* , Time Books, Random House, NY

Chapter Seven--Telling the Truth

1 - According to the American Academy of Cosmetic Surgery

2 - In 1994, two million prescriptions per month were written for Prozac and that number has been rising since.

3 - If you are interested in this science known as psycho-neuro-immunology, I recommend any books written by Joan Borysenko or Bernie Siegel.

4 - Sogyal Rinpoche, *The Tibetan Book of Living and Dying*, Harper San Francisco, 1992, pg. 57

ORDER FORM

To order additional copies of
Kiss Your Fat Good-Bye
send a check or money order for
$12.95 plus $2.OO for postage
per book to:

Aroha Press
63366 Saddleback Pl.
Bend Or 97701
541-385-9465

....

SEND TO:

Name:_____

Address:_____

City, State, Zip: _____

Phone Number:_____

Number of books:_____

Total amount enclosed:_____